ATS-75   ADMISSION TEST SERIES

This is your
PASSBOOK for...

NCLEX-RN

National Council Licensure Examination for Registered Nurses

Test Preparation Study Guide
Questions & Answers

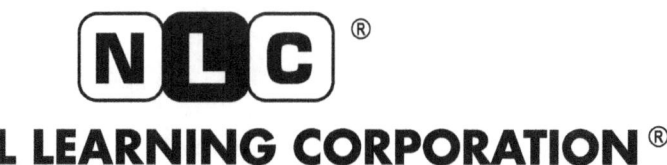

COPYRIGHT NOTICE

This book is SOLELY intended for, is sold ONLY to, and its use is RESTRICTED to individual, bona fide applicants or candidates who qualify by virtue of having seriously filed applications for appropriate license, certificate, professional and/or promotional advancement, higher school matriculation, scholarship, or other legitimate requirements of education and/or governmental authorities.

This book is NOT intended for use, class instruction, tutoring, training, duplication, copying, reprinting, excerption, or adaptation, etc., by:

1) Other publishers
2) Proprietors and/or Instructors of "Coaching" and/or Preparatory Courses
3) Personnel and/or Training Divisions of commercial, industrial, and governmental organizations
4) Schools, colleges, or universities and/or their departments and staffs, including teachers and other personnel
5) Testing Agencies or Bureaus
6) Study groups which seek by the purchase of a single volume to copy and/or duplicate and/or adapt this material for use by the group as a whole without having purchased individual volumes for each of the members of the group
7) Et al.

Such persons would be in violation of appropriate Federal and State statutes.

PROVISION OF LICENSING AGREEMENTS – Recognized educational, commercial, industrial, and governmental institutions and organizations, and others legitimately engaged in educational pursuits, including training, testing, and measurement activities, may address request for a licensing agreement to the copyright owners, who will determine whether, and under what conditions, including fees and charges, the materials in this book may be used them. In other words, a licensing facility exists for the legitimate use of the material in this book on other than an individual basis. However, it is asseverated and affirmed here that the material in this book CANNOT be used without the receipt of the express permission of such a licensing agreement from the Publishers. Inquiries re licensing should be addressed to the company, attention rights and permissions department.

All rights reserved, including the right of reproduction in whole or in part, in any form or by any means, electronic or mechanical, including photocopying, recording, or by any information storage and retrieval system, without permission in writing from the Publisher.

Copyright © 2024 by
National Learning Corporation

212 Michael Drive, Syosset, NY 11791
(516) 921-8888 • www.passbooks.com
E-mail: info@passbooks.com

PASSBOOK® SERIES

THE *PASSBOOK® SERIES* has been created to prepare applicants and candidates for the ultimate academic battlefield – the examination room.

At some time in our lives, each and every one of us may be required to take an examination – for validation, matriculation, admission, qualification, registration, certification, or licensure.

Based on the assumption that every applicant or candidate has met the basic formal educational standards, has taken the required number of courses, and read the necessary texts, the *PASSBOOK® SERIES* furnishes the one special preparation which may assure passing with confidence, instead of failing with insecurity. Examination questions – together with answers – are furnished as the basic vehicle for study so that the mysteries of the examination and its compounding difficulties may be eliminated or diminished by a sure method.

This book is meant to help you pass your examination provided that you qualify and are serious in your objective.

The entire field is reviewed through the huge store of content information which is succinctly presented through a provocative and challenging approach – the question-and-answer method.

A climate of success is established by furnishing the correct answers at the end of each test.

You soon learn to recognize types of questions, forms of questions, and patterns of questioning. You may even begin to anticipate expected outcomes.

You perceive that many questions are repeated or adapted so that you can gain acute insights, which may enable you to score many sure points.

You learn how to confront new questions, or types of questions, and to attack them confidently and work out the correct answers.

You note objectives and emphases, and recognize pitfalls and dangers, so that you may make positive educational adjustments.

Moreover, you are kept fully informed in relation to new concepts, methods, practices, and directions in the field.

You discover that you are actually taking the examination all the time: you are preparing for the examination by "taking" an examination, not by reading extraneous and/or supererogatory textbooks.

In short, this PASSBOOK®, used directedly, should be an important factor in helping you to pass your test.

Introduction

ABOUT THE NCLEX-RN

This book has been designed to assist you in preparing for the licensure examination which you must take to become a registered nurse in the United States. For purposes of this book, states are defined to include the United States, the District of Columbia, Guam and the Virgin Islands. In all 53 states, candidates take the National Council Licensure Examinations (NCLEX) as a part of the process of becoming eligible for licensure as registered nurses.

Until 1982, the test was called the State Board Test Pool Examination for Registered Nurse Licensure, abbreviated SBTPE. The National Council of State Boards of Nursing, the organization that prepares the exams, has changed the name of the exam to NCLEX, standing for National Council Licensure Examinations. The RN and LPN examinations are called NCLEX-RN and NCLEX-PN. The exams are required of all nursing candidates, and they are intended to determine whether or not you are prepared to practice nursing safely.

The first section of this book provides a general introduction to the examination. You will be given specific information on how to prepare for and take the examination.

Entry to the practice of nursing is regulated by law for the protection of the public. Boards of nursing exist in all the states and territories of the United States, and as a nurse-to-be you must provide the nursing board in your state with evidence of your ability to deliver effective nursing care. The licensure examinations were developed to test for safe and effective nursing practice. The individual boards of nursing organized the National Council of State Boards of Nursing as a central membership organization.

The examination tests your ability to apply knowledge of nursing by asking questions about health care situations demanding nursing intervention. It is designed to test essential knowledge in nursing and to make certain that you have the ability to apply that knowledge in clinical situations.

The two-day examination is usually given twice a year in February and July. All participating states administer the examination on the same dates although in sites selected separately by each state. Each state agency sets up its own cut-off date for applying for admission to the examination and has an application process that must be followed. You must request admission to the licensure examination by contacting the state board of nursing of the state in which you wish to be licensed.

The examination is composed of questions that test nursing knowledge. As a candidate for licensure, you have completed a course of instruction in a degree-granting or diploma-granting program or have completed a series of competency tests. During the educational process, you have learned nursing through study, classroom activities, and clinical practice. The basic information necessary to give safe and effective nursing is determined by the faculty of the school, who select essential material to be learned.

HOW TO PREPARE FOR THE EXAMINATION

The NCLEX is intended to measure the abilities required for nursing practice. What you have learned in nursing school to prepare you for practice should provide the necessary preparation for taking the NCLEX.

Most candidates will probably want to do some reviewing in preparation for the NCLEX, and this is appropriate. The best preparation is likely to consist of a review of the text books and class notes that you used in nursing school combined with intensive study and practice from this book.

The conditions described in the NCLEX consist of common health problems. However, even if you have never heard of the condition described, you should be able to get many right answers by applying general principles. For example, the principles of asepsis apply to all patients with wounds or incisions; they don't depend on the specific nature of a wound or incision considered in a situation. In most cases, the general principle will lead you to the correct answer. Therefore, if you have not had the experience with a situation that appears on the test, but you have had experience with similar situations, you can answer questions on the basis of such similarity.

There is a practical difference between clinical nursing and test taking. In nursing practice, you should not act on the basis of partial information, vague similarities, and guesses. However, on a test you should indicate what you know, and the fact that your knowledge is incomplete should not stop you from analyzing the question and applying your best judgment. In some cases, your knowledge and judgment may be more complete than you suspect.

HOW THE TEST IS SCORED

The examination is given in four parts, called Books I,II,III, and IV, for ease in administering the exam and to provide a break every two hours. But these parts do not differ from each other in subject area covered, and the exam is given a single score. If you fail, you must re-take the entire examination in order to pass. Scores range from 800 up to about 3200. The recommended passing score is 1600. The pass rate for first-time candidates is approximately 85 percent. No points are subtracted for wrong answers, and it will be entirely to your advantage to go ahead and guess on questions you do not know.

SCOPE OF THE EXAMINATION

The test plan is comprised of nursing behaviors, systems of client health requirements and levels of cognitive ability.

NURSING BEHAVIORS

Nursing behaviors to be tested are grouped under the broad categories of assessing, analyzing, planning, implementing and evaluating. The nurse collects data about the client, identifies specific needs, plans with the client and/or significant others to meet those needs, implements a plan of care and evaluates the effects of the intervention. Because the five categories have equal importance, each one is assigned approximately 20 percent of the total items in the examination

SYSTEMS OF CLIENT HEALTH REQUIREMENTS

The health requirements of clients are defined within systems that are designated in relation to the locus of decision making and the scope of care to be provided. Situations are drawn from all types of client-nurse interaction.

The systems are described as follows:

1. The locus of decision making is centered in the nurse when clients are unable to make decisions regarding their physical and/or psychological status. These clients are in life-threatening situations that require therapeutic intervention.

2. The locus of decision making is shared by the nurse and the client when the latter is able to exercise partial control in meeting health requirements and to perform selected activities of daily living. These clients are in situations that require a therapeutic regimen to maintain life or improve health.

3. The locus of decision making is centered in clients when they are able to manage their health care needs independently. These clients are in situations that require education for promotion of health, guidance or support for prevention of disease, and/or provision of an environment for growth.

    Twenty or thirty percent of the test items will reflect the system in which the locus of decision making is centered in the nurse; 55 to 65 percent, the system in which the locus of decision making is shared by the client and nurse; and 10 to 20 percent, the system in which the locus of decision making is centered in the client

LEVELS OF COGNITIVE ABILITY

The examination includes test items at the cognitive levels of knowledge, comprehension, application and analysis. Weighting is not specified for the levels of cognitive ability; however, most items in the examination are at the application and analysis levels.

SPECIFIC NURSING BEHAVIORS TO BE MEASURED IN THE EXAMINATION FOR LICENSURE

I. Assessing; establishing a data base about a client.

   A. Gathers information relative to the client.
      1. Collects information from verbal interactions with client, family and/or significant others.
      2. Examines standard data sources for information.
      3. Recognizes symptoms and findings.
      4. Determines client's ability to assume care of daily health needs.
      5. Assesses environment of client.
      6. Identifies own or staff reactions to client, client's family or significant others.

B. Verifies data.
1. Confirms observation or perception by obtaining additional information.
2. Questions orders and decisions by other staff when indicated.
3. Checks conditions of client personally instead of relying upon equipment.

C. Communicates information gained in assessment of client.

II. Analyzing: identifying the client's health care needs and selecting goals of care.

A. Interprets data.

B. Identifies client needs.

C. Determines goals of care.
1. Involves client, family and significant others in setting goals.
2. Establishes priorities among goals.
3. Projects expected outcomes of nursing intervention.

III. Planning: designing a strategy to achieve the goals established for client care.

A. Develops and modifies client care plan.
1. Anticipates needs of client on basis of established priorities.
2. Involves the client and/or family in designing the strategy for care.
3. Includes all information needed for managing the client's condition, such as age,
4. sex, culture, ethnicity and religion.
5. Plans for client's comfort and maintenance of optimal functioning.
6. Selects nursing measures for delivery of client care.

B. Cooperates with other health personnel for delivery of client care.
1. Coordinates care for benefit of client.
2. Identifies health or social resources in the community for client and/or family.

C. Records information relevant to client management.

IV. IV. Implementing: initiating and completing actions necessary to accomplish the defined goals.

A. Performs or assists in performing activities of daily living.
1. Institutes measures for client's comfort.
2. Assists client to maintain optimal functioning.

B. Counsels and teaches client and/or family.
1. Helps client and/or family to recognize and manage psychological stress.
2. Facilitates relationships of family, staff or significant others with client.
3. Teaches correct principles, procedures and techniques of health care.
4. Informs client about his health status.
5. Refers client and/or family to appropriate health or social resources in the community.

C. Gives care to achieve therapeutic goals for the client.
   1. Institutes action to compensate for adverse reactions.
   2. Uses precautionary and preventive measures in giving care to client.
   3. Uses correct techniques in administering client care.
   4. Prepares client for surgery, delivery or other procedures.
   5. Initiates necessary life-saving measures for emergency situations.

D. Gives care to optimize achievement of health goals by the client.
   1. Provides an environment conducive to attainment of client's health care goals.
   2. Adjusts care in accord with client's expressed or implied needs.
   3. Stimulates and motivates client, enabling him to achieve self care and independence.
   4. Encourages client to accept care or adhere to treatment regime.
   5. Compensates for own and staff reactions to factors influencing therapeutic relationships with clients.

E. Supervises and checks the work of staff for whom responsible.

F. Records and exchanges information.
   1. Gives complete, accurate reports on assigned clients to other team members.
   2. Records nursing actions and other information relevant to implementation of care.

V. Evaluating: determining the extent to which the goals of care have been achieved.

A. Estimates the extent to which objectives of the plan of care are achieved.
   1. Recognizes effects (intended and unintended) of measures used.
   2. Determines if there is a need to change goals established for client care.

B. Evaluates implementation of measures.
   1. Judges accuracy of implementation of measures.
   2. Determines if there is a need for change in the environment, equipment or procedures.

C. Investigates compliance with prescribed and/or proscribed therapy.
   1. Judges impact of actions on client, family and staff.
   2. Checks to insure that tests or measurements are done correctly.
   3. Ascertains client's and/or family's understanding of information or care given.

D. Records client's response to treatment or care.

HOW TO TAKE A TEST

You have studied long, hard and conscientiously.

With your official admission card in hand, and your heart pounding, you have been admitted to the examination room.

You note that there are several hundred other applicants in the examination room waiting to take the same test.

They all appear to be equally well prepared.

You know that nothing but your best effort will suffice. The "moment of truth" is at hand: you now have to demonstrate objectively, in writing, your knowledge of content and your understanding of subject matter.

You are fighting the most important battle of your life—to pass and/or score high on an examination which will determine your career and provide the economic basis for your livelihood.

What extra, special things should you know and should you do in taking the examination?

I. YOU MUST PASS AN EXAMINATION

A. WHAT EVERY CANDIDATE SHOULD KNOW
   Examination applicants often ask us for help in preparing for the written test. What can I study in advance? What kinds of questions will be asked? How will the test be given? How will the papers be graded?

B. HOW ARE EXAMS DEVELOPED?
   Examinations are carefully written by trained technicians who are specialists in the field known as "psychological measurement," in consultation with recognized authorities in the field of work that the test will cover. These experts recommend the subject matter areas or skills to be tested; only those knowledges or skills important to your success on the job are included. The most reliable books and source materials available are used as references. Together, the experts and technicians judge the difficulty level of the questions.
   Test technicians know how to phrase questions so that the problem is clearly stated. Their ethics do not permit "trick" or "catch" questions. Questions may have been tried out on sample groups, or subjected to statistical analysis, to determine their usefulness.
   Written tests are often used in combination with performance tests, ratings of training and experience, and oral interviews. All of these measures combine to form the best-known means of finding the right person for the right job.

II. HOW TO PASS THE WRITTEN TEST

A. BASIC STEPS

1) Study the announcement

How, then, can you know what subjects to study? Our best answer is: "Learn as much as possible about the class of positions for which you've applied." The exam will test the knowledge, skills and abilities needed to do the work.

Your most valuable source of information about the position you want is the official exam announcement. This announcement lists the training and experience qualifications. Check these standards and apply only if you come reasonably close to meeting them. Many jurisdictions preview the written test in the exam announcement by including a section called "Knowledge and Abilities Required," "Scope of the Examination," or some similar heading. Here you will find out specifically what fields will be tested.

2) Choose appropriate study materials

If the position for which you are applying is technical or advanced, you will read more advanced, specialized material. If you are already familiar with the basic principles of your field, elementary textbooks would waste your time. Concentrate on advanced textbooks and technical periodicals. Think through the concepts and review difficult problems in your field.

These are all general sources. You can get more ideas on your own initiative, following these leads. For example, training manuals and publications of the government agency which employs workers in your field can be useful, particularly for technical and professional positions. A letter or visit to the government department involved may result in more specific study suggestions, and certainly will provide you with a more definite idea of the exact nature of the position you are seeking.

3) Study this book!

III. KINDS OF TESTS

Tests are used for purposes other than measuring knowledge and ability to perform specified duties. For some positions, it is equally important to test ability to make adjustments to new situations or to profit from training. In others, basic mental abilities not dependent on information are essential. Questions which test these things may not appear as pertinent to the duties of the position as those which test for knowledge and information. Yet they are often highly important parts of a fair examination. For very general questions, it is almost impossible to help you direct your study efforts. What we can do is to point out some of the more common of these general abilities needed in public service positions and describe some typical questions.

1) General information

Broad, general information has been found useful for predicting job success in some kinds of work. This is tested in a variety of ways, from vocabulary lists to questions about current events. Basic background in some field of work, such as sociology or economics, may be sampled in a group of questions. Often these are principles which have become familiar to most persons through exposure rather than through formal training. It is difficult to advise you how to study for these questions; being alert to the world around you is our best suggestion.

2) Verbal ability

An example of an ability needed in many positions is verbal or language ability. Verbal ability is, in brief, the ability to use and understand words. Vocabulary and grammar tests are typical measures of this ability. Reading comprehension or paragraph interpretation questions are common in many kinds of civil service tests. You are given a paragraph of written material and asked to find its central meaning.

IV. KINDS OF QUESTIONS

1. Multiple-choice Questions

Most popular of the short-answer questions is the "multiple choice" or "best answer" question. It can be used, for example, to test for factual knowledge, ability to solve problems or judgment in meeting situations found at work.

A multiple-choice question is normally one of three types:
- It can begin with an incomplete statement followed by several possible endings. You are to find the one ending which best completes the statement, although some of the others may not be entirely wrong.
- It can also be a complete statement in the form of a question which is answered by choosing one of the statements listed.
- It can be in the form of a problem – again you select the best answer.

Here is an example of a multiple-choice question with a discussion which should give you some clues as to the method for choosing the right answer:

When an employee has a complaint about his assignment, the action which will best help him overcome his difficulty is to
- A. discuss his difficulty with his coworkers
- B. take the problem to the head of the organization
- C. take the problem to the person who gave him the assignment
- D. say nothing to anyone about his complaint

In answering this question, you should study each of the choices to find which is best. Consider choice "A" – Certainly an employee may discuss his complaint with fellow employees, but no change or improvement can result, and the complaint remains unresolved. Choice "B" is a poor choice since the head of the organization probably does not know what assignment you have been given, and taking your problem to him is known as "going over the head" of the supervisor. The supervisor, or person who made the assignment, is the person who can clarify it or correct any injustice. Choice "C" is, therefore, correct. To say nothing, as in choice "D," is unwise. Supervisors have and interest in knowing the problems employees are facing, and the employee is seeking a solution to his problem.

2. True/False

3. Matching Questions

Matching an answer from a column of choices within another column.

V. RECORDING YOUR ANSWERS

Computer terminals are used more and more today for many different kinds of exams.

For an examination with very few applicants, you may be told to record your answers in the test booklet itself. Separate answer sheets are much more common. If this separate answer sheet is to be scored by machine – and this is often the case – it is highly important that you mark your answers correctly in order to get credit.

VI. BEFORE THE TEST

YOUR PHYSICAL CONDITION IS IMPORTANT

If you are not well, you can't do your best work on tests. If you are half asleep, you can't do your best either. Here are some tips:

1) Get about the same amount of sleep you usually get. Don't stay up all night before the test, either partying or worrying—DON'T DO IT!
2) If you wear glasses, be sure to wear them when you go to take the test. This goes for hearing aids, too.
3) If you have any physical problems that may keep you from doing your best, be sure to tell the person giving the test. If you are sick or in poor health, you relay cannot do your best on any test. You can always come back and take the test some other time.

Common sense will help you find procedures to follow to get ready for an examination. Too many of us, however, overlook these sensible measures. Indeed, nervousness and fatigue have been found to be the most serious reasons why applicants fail to do their best on civil service tests. Here is a list of reminders:

- Begin your preparation early – Don't wait until the last minute to go scurrying around for books and materials or to find out what the position is all about.
- Prepare continuously – An hour a night for a week is better than an all-night cram session. This has been definitely established. What is more, a night a week for a month will return better dividends than crowding your study into a shorter period of time.
- Locate the place of the exam – You have been sent a notice telling you when and where to report for the examination. If the location is in a different town or otherwise unfamiliar to you, it would be well to inquire the best route and learn something about the building.
- Relax the night before the test – Allow your mind to rest. Do not study at all that night. Plan some mild recreation or diversion; then go to bed early and get a good night's sleep.
- Get up early enough to make a leisurely trip to the place for the test – This way unforeseen events, traffic snarls, unfamiliar buildings, etc. will not upset you.
- Dress comfortably – A written test is not a fashion show. You will be known by number and not by name, so wear something comfortable.
- Leave excess paraphernalia at home – Shopping bags and odd bundles will get in your way. You need bring only the items mentioned in the official notice you received; usually everything you need is provided. Do not bring reference books to the exam. They will only confuse those last minutes and be taken away from you when in the test room.

- Arrive somewhat ahead of time – If because of transportation schedules you must get there very early, bring a newspaper or magazine to take your mind off yourself while waiting.
- Locate the examination room – When you have found the proper room, you will be directed to the seat or part of the room where you will sit. Sometimes you are given a sheet of instructions to read while you are waiting. Do not fill out any forms until you are told to do so; just read them and be prepared.
- Relax and prepare to listen to the instructions
- If you have any physical problem that may keep you from doing your best, be sure to tell the test administrator. If you are sick or in poor health, you really cannot do your best on the exam. You can come back and take the test some other time.

VII. AT THE TEST

The day of the test is here and you have the test booklet in your hand. The temptation to get going is very strong. Caution! There is more to success than knowing the right answers. You must know how to identify your papers and understand variations in the type of short-answer question used in this particular examination. Follow these suggestions for maximum results from your efforts:

1) Cooperate with the monitor

The test administrator has a duty to create a situation in which you can be as much at ease as possible. He will give instructions, tell you when to begin, check to see that you are marking your answer sheet correctly, and so on. He is not there to guard you, although he will see that your competitors do not take unfair advantage. He wants to help you do your best.

2) Listen to all instructions

Don't jump the gun! Wait until you understand all directions. In most civil service tests you get more time than you need to answer the questions. So don't be in a hurry. Read each word of instructions until you clearly understand the meaning. Study the examples, listen to all announcements and follow directions. Ask questions if you do not understand what to do.

3) Identify your papers

Civil service exams are usually identified by number only. You will be assigned a number; you must not put your name on your test papers. Be sure to copy your number correctly. Since more than one exam may be given, copy your exact examination title.

4) Plan your time

Unless you are told that a test is a "speed" or "rate of work" test, speed itself is usually not important. Time enough to answer all the questions will be provided, but this does not mean that you have all day. An overall time limit has been set. Divide the total time (in minutes) by the number of questions to determine the approximate time you have for each question.

5) Do not linger over difficult questions

If you come across a difficult question, mark it with a paper clip (useful to have along) and come back to it when you have been through the booklet. One caution if you do this – be sure to skip a number on your answer sheet as well. Check often to be sure that you have not lost your place and that you are marking in the row numbered the same as the question you are answering.

6) Read the questions

Be sure you know what the question asks! Many capable people are unsuccessful because they failed to read the questions correctly.

7) Answer all questions

Unless you have been instructed that a penalty will be deducted for incorrect answers, it is better to guess than to omit a question.

8) Speed tests

It is often better NOT to guess on speed tests. It has been found that on timed tests people are tempted to spend the last few seconds before time is called in marking answers at random – without even reading them – in the hope of picking up a few extra points. To discourage this practice, the instructions may warn you that your score will be "corrected" for guessing. That is, a penalty will be applied. The incorrect answers will be deducted from the correct ones, or some other penalty formula will be used.

9) Review your answers

If you finish before time is called, go back to the questions you guessed or omitted to give them further thought. Review other answers if you have time.

10) Return your test materials

If you are ready to leave before others have finished or time is called, take ALL your materials to the monitor and leave quietly. Never take any test material with you. The monitor can discover whose papers are not complete, and taking a test booklet may be grounds for disqualification.

VIII. EXAMINATION TECHNIQUES

1) Read the general instructions carefully. These are usually printed on the first page of the exam booklet. As a rule, these instructions refer to the timing of the examination; the fact that you should not start work until the signal and must stop work at a signal, etc. If there are any special instructions, such as a choice of questions to be answered, make sure that you note this instruction carefully.

2) When you are ready to start work on the examination, that is as soon as the signal has been given, read the instructions to each question booklet, underline any key words or phrases, such as least, best, outline, describe and the like. In this way you will tend to answer as requested rather than discover on reviewing your paper that you listed without describing, that you selected the worst choice rather than the best choice, etc.

3) If the examination is of the objective or multiple-choice type – that is, each question will also give a series of possible answers: A, B, C or D, and you are called upon to select the best answer and write the letter next to that answer on your answer paper – it is advisable to start answering each question in turn. There may be anywhere from 50 to 100 such questions in the three or four hours allotted and you can see how much time would be taken if you read through all the questions before beginning to answer any. Furthermore, if you

come across a question or group of questions which you know would be difficult to answer, it would undoubtedly affect your handling of all the other questions.

4) If the examination is of the essay type and contains but a few questions, it is a moot point as to whether you should read all the questions before starting to answer any one. Of course, if you are given a choice – say five out of seven and the like – then it is essential to read all the questions so you can eliminate the two that are most difficult. If, however, you are asked to answer all the questions, there may be danger in trying to answer the easiest one first because you may find that you will spend too much time on it. The best technique is to answer the first question, then proceed to the second, etc.

5) Time your answers. Before the exam begins, write down the time it started, then add the time allowed for the examination and write down the time it must be completed, then divide the time available somewhat as follows:
    - If 3-1/2 hours are allowed, that would be 210 minutes. If you have 80 objective-type questions, that would be an average of 2-1/2 minutes per question. Allow yourself no more than 2 minutes per question, or a total of 160 minutes, which will permit about 50 minutes to review.
    - If for the time allotment of 210 minutes there are 7 essay questions to answer, that would average about 30 minutes a question. Give yourself only 25 minutes per question so that you have about 35 minutes to review.

6) The most important instruction is to read each question and make sure you know what is wanted. The second most important instruction is to time yourself properly so that you answer every question. The third most important instruction is to answer every question. Guess if you have to but include something for each question. Remember that you will receive no credit for a blank and will probably receive some credit if you write something in answer to an essay question. If you guess a letter – say "B" for a multiple-choice question – you may have guessed right. If you leave a blank as an answer to a multiple-choice question, the examiners may respect your feelings but it will not add a point to your score. Some exams may penalize you for wrong answers, so in such cases only, you may not want to guess unless you have some basis for your answer.

7) Suggestions
    a. Objective-type questions
        1. Examine the question booklet for proper sequence of pages and questions
        2. Read all instructions carefully
        3. Skip any question which seems too difficult; return to it after all other questions have been answered
        4. Apportion your time properly; do not spend too much time on any single question or group of questions
        5. Note and underline key words – all, most, fewest, least, best, worst, same, opposite, etc.
        6. Pay particular attention to negatives
        7. Note unusual option, e.g., unduly long, short, complex, different or similar in content to the body of the question
        8. Observe the use of "hedging" words – probably, may, most likely, etc.

9. Make sure that your answer is put next to the same number as the question
10. Do not second-guess unless you have good reason to believe the second answer is definitely more correct
11. Cross out original answer if you decide another answer is more accurate; do not erase until you are ready to hand your paper in
12. Answer all questions; guess unless instructed otherwise
13. Leave time for review

b. Essay questions
1. Read each question carefully
2. Determine exactly what is wanted. Underline key words or phrases.
3. Decide on outline or paragraph answer
4. Include many different points and elements unless asked to develop any one or two points or elements
5. Show impartiality by giving pros and cons unless directed to select one side only
6. Make and write down any assumptions you find necessary to answer the questions
7. Watch your English, grammar, punctuation and choice of words
8. Time your answers; don't crowd material

8) Answering the essay question

Most essay questions can be answered by framing the specific response around several key words or ideas. Here are a few such key words or ideas:

M's: manpower, materials, methods, money, management
P's: purpose, program, policy, plan, procedure, practice, problems, pitfalls, personnel, public relations

a. Six basic steps in handling problems:
1. Preliminary plan and background development
2. Collect information, data and facts
3. Analyze and interpret information, data and facts
4. Analyze and develop solutions as well as make recommendations
5. Prepare report and sell recommendations
6. Install recommendations and follow up effectiveness

b. Pitfalls to avoid
1. Taking things for granted – A statement of the situation does not necessarily imply that each of the elements is necessarily true; for example, a complaint may be invalid and biased so that all that can be taken for granted is that a complaint has been registered
2. Considering only one side of a situation – Wherever possible, indicate several alternatives and then point out the reasons you selected the best one
3. Failing to indicate follow up – Whenever your answer indicates action on your part, make certain that you will take proper follow-up action to see how successful your recommendations, procedures or actions turn out to be
4. Taking too long in answering any single question – Remember to time your answers properly

EXAMINATION SECTION

EXAMINATION SECTION
TEST 1

DIRECTIONS: Each question or incomplete statement is followed by several suggested answers or completions. Select the one that BEST answers the question or completes the statement. *PRINT THE LETTER OF THE CORRECT ANSWER IN THE SPACE AT THE RIGHT.*

1. The abbreviation *EEG* refers to a(n) 1.____

    A. examination of the eyes and ears
    B. inflammatory disease of the urinogenital tract
    C. disease of the esophogeal structure
    D. examination of the brain

2. The complete destruction of all forms of living microorganisms is called 2.____

    A. decontamination   B. fumigation
    C. sterilization   D. germination

3. A rectal thermometer differs from other fever thermometers in that it has a 3.____

    A. longer stem   B. thinner stem
    C. stubby bulb at one end D. slender bulb at one end

4. The one of the following pieces of equipment which is USUALLY used together with a sphygmometer is a 4.____

    A. stethoscope   B. watch
    C. fever thermometer   D. hypodermic syringe

5. A curette is a 5.____

    A. healing drug   B. curved scalpel
    C. long hypodermic needle D. scraping instrument

6. The otoscope is used to examine the patient's 6.____

    A. eyes   B. ears   C. mouth   D. lungs

7. A catheter is used 7.____

    A. to close wounds
    B. for withdrawing fluid from a body cavity
    C. to remove cataracts
    D. as a cathartic

8. Of the following pieces of equipment, the one that is required for making a scratch test is a 8.____

    A. needle   B. scalpel
    C. capillary tube D. tourniquet

9. A hemostat is an instrument which is used to

   A. hold a sterile needle
   B. clamp off a blood vessel
   C. regulate the temperature of a sterilizer
   D. measure oxygen intake

10. Of the following medical supplies, the one that MUST be stored in a tightly sealed bottle is

    A. sodium fluoride
    B. alum
    C. oil of cloves
    D. aromatic spirits of ammonia

11. A person who has been exposed to an infectious disease is called

    A. a contact   B. an incubator
    C. diseased   D. infected

12. A myocardial infarct would occur in the

    A. heart   B. kidneys   C. lungs   D. spleen

13. The abbreviations *WBC* and *RBC* refer to the results of tests of the

    A. basal metabolism   B. blood
    C. blood pressure   D. bony structure

14. When a person's blood pressure is noted as 120/80, it means that his _____ blood pressure is _____.

    A. pulse; 120   B. pulse; 80
    C. systolic; 120   D. systolic; 80

15. The anatomical structure that contains the tonsils and adenoids is the

    A. pharynx   B. larynx   C. trachea   D. sinuses

16. An abscess can BEST be described as a

    A. loss of sensation   B. painful tooth
    C. ruptured membrane   D. localized formation of pus

17. Nephritis is a disease affecting the

    A. gall bladder   B. larynx
    C. kidney   D. large intestine

18. Hemoglobin is contained in the

    A. white blood cells   B. lymph fluids
    C. platelets   D. red blood cells

19. Bile is a body fluid that is MOST directly concerned with

    A. digestion   B. excretion
    C. reproduction   D. metabolism

20. Of the following bones, the one which is located below the waist is the   20.____

    A. sternum   B. clavicle   C. tibia   D. humerus

21. The one of the following which is NOT part of the digestive canal is the   21.____

    A. esophagus   B. larynx   C. duodenum   D. colon

22. The thyroid and the pituitary are part of the _____ system.   22.____

    A. digestive   B. endocrine
    C. respiratory   D. excretory

23. The one of the following which would be included in a *GU* examination is the   23.____

    A. rectum   B. trachea   C. kidneys   D. pancreas

24. Of the following, the one which would be included in the x-ray examination known as a *GI series* is the   24.____

    A. colon   B. skull   C. lungs   D. uterus

25. A person who, while not ill himself, may transmit a disease to another person is known as a(n)   25.____

    A. breeder   B. incubator   C. carrier   D. inhibitor

KEY (CORRECT ANSWERS)

1. D
2. C
3. C
4. A
5. D

6. B
7. B
8. A
9. B
10. D

11. A
12. A
13. B
14. C
15. A

16. D
17. C
18. D
19. A
20. C

21. B
22. B
23. C
24. A
25. D

TEST 2

DIRECTIONS: Each question or incomplete statement is followed by several suggested answers or completions. Select the one that BEST answers the question or completes the statement. *PRINT THE LETTER OF THE CORRECT ANSWER IN THE SPACE AT THE RIGHT.*

1. Thorough washing of the hands for two minutes with soap and warm water will leave the hands   1.___

    A. sterile
    B. aseptic
    C. decontaminated
    D. partially disinfected

2. The one of the following which is BEST for preparing the skin for an injection is   2.___

    A. green soap and water
    B. alcohol
    C. phenol
    D. formalin

3. A fever thermometer should be cleansed after use by washing it with   3.___

    A. soap and cool water
    B. warm water *only*
    C. soap and hot water
    D. running cold tap water

4. The FIRST step in cleaning an instrument which has fresh blood on it is to   4.___

    A. wash it in hot soapy water
    B. soak it in a boric acid bath
    C. wash it under cool running water
    D. soak it in 70% alcohol

5. If a contaminated nasal speculum cannot be sterilized immediately after use, then the BEST procedure to follow until sterilization is possible is to place it   5.___

    A. under a piece of dry gauze
    B. in warm water
    C. in alcohol
    D. in a green soap solution

6. A hypodermic needle should ALWAYS be checked to see if it has a good sharp point   6.___

    A. when it is being washed
    B. when it is removed from the sterilizer
    C. just before it is sterilized
    D. immediately before an injection

7. Of the following, the LOWEST temperature at which cotton goods will be sterilized, if placed in an autoclave for 30 minutes, is   7.___

    A. 130° F   B. 170° F   C. 200° F   D. 250° F

8. Of the following procedures, the one which is BEST for sterilizing an ear speculum which is contaminated with wax is to   8.___

A. scrub it with cold soapy water, rinse in ether, and place in boiling water for 20 minutes
B. soak it in warm water, scrub in cold soapy water, rinse with water, and autoclave at 275° F for 10 minutes
C. wash it in alcohol, scrub in hot soapy water, rinse with water, and place in boiling water for 20 minutes
D. wash it in 1% Lysol solution, rinse, and autoclave at 275° F for 15 minutes

9. Assume that clean water accidentally spilled on the outside of a package of cloth-wrapped hypodermic syringes which has been sterilized.
Of the following, the BEST action to take is to

9.____

A. leave the package to dry in a sunny, clean place
B. sterilize the package again
C. remove the wet cloth and wrap the package in a dry sterile cloth
D. wipe off the package with a clean dry towel and later ask the nurse in charge what to do

10. Hypodermic needles should be sterilized by placing them in

10.____

A. boiling water for 5 minutes
B. an autoclave at 15 lbs. pressure for 15 minutes
C. oil heated to 220° F for 10 minutes
D. a 1:40 Lysol solution for 10 minutes

11. A cutting instrument should be sterilized by placing it in

11.____

A. a chemical germicide
B. an autoclave at 15 lbs. pressure for 20 minutes
C. boiling water for 20 minutes
D. a hot air oven at 320° F for 1 hour

12. A fever thermometer used by a patient who has tuberculosis should be washed and then placed in

12.____

A. boiling water for 10 minutes
B. a hot air oven for 20 minutes
C. a 1:1000 solution of bichloride of mercury for one minute
D. an autoclave at 15 lbs. pressure for 15 minutes

13. The MOST reliable method of sterilizing a glass syringe is to place it in

13.____

A. Zephiran chloride 1:1000 solution for 40 minutes
B. oil heated to 250° F for 12 minutes
C. boiling water for 20 minutes
D. an autoclave at 15 lbs. pressure for 20 minutes

14. The insides of sterilizers should be cleaned daily with a mild abrasive PRIMARILY to

14.____

A. remove scale
B. prevent the growth of bacteria
C. remove blood and other organic matter
D. prevent acids from damaging the sterilizer

15. Of the following, the BEST reason for giving a patient a jar in which to bring a urine specimen on his next visit to the clinic is that the

    A. patient may not have a jar at home
    B. patient may bring the specimen in a jar which is too large
    C. patient may bring the specimen in a jar which has not been cleaned properly
    D. jar may be misplaced if it is not a jar in which urine specimens are usually collected

16. Simply providing nutritional information and recommended low-cost diets to clinic patients has not resulted in improved diets for their children.
    The MOST plausible conclusion to draw from this statement is that

    A. nutrition is only one factor in improving health
    B. nutrition is of greater value in improving the health of adults than in improving the health of children
    C. the health problems of clinic patients are not caused by nutritional defects
    D. clinic patients are not using the nutritional information given them

17. Many people who appear to be robust are highly susceptible to disease and are outlived by many seemingly frail people. Of the following, the MOST plausible conclusion which may be drawn from this statement is that

    A. physical appearance is not a reliable indicator of health
    B. frail people take better care of themselves than do robust people
    C. disease tends to strike robust people more frequently than frail people
    D. robust people tend to overexert themselves more often than frail people do

18. The skill of interviewers, the wording of questions, and the willingness of patients to respond freely to questions all affect the results of a survey. Reports of surveys of patient attitudes toward the health work of the clinic are therefore valueless unless we also know how the surveys were conducted. A recent report that 85% of clinic patients were satisfied with clinic service must be treated with caution; it may be that another survey would have revealed just the opposite!
    On the basis of this paragraph, it is MOST accurate to conclude that

    A. survey reports have little value in determining patient attitudes
    B. contrary to a recent report, 85% of clinic patients are dissatisfied with clinic service
    C. published results of surveys may be misleading unless accompanied by knowledge of the methods used
    D. listening to the unsolicited comments of clinic patients is of greater value than questioning them directly concerning their attitudes

Questions 19-25.

DIRECTIONS: Questions 19 through 25 are to be answered on the basis of the following table.

STATISTICAL REPORT ON CLINICS IN XYZ HEALTH CENTER, AUGUST				
	APPOINTMENTS		PROCEDURES	
CLINIC	NO. OF APPOINTMENTS SCHEDULE	NO. OF BROKEN APPOINTMENTS	NO. OF DIAGNOSTIC PROCEDURES	NO. OF SURGICAL PROCEDURES
A	1400	260	1910	140
B	730	160	2000	500
C	1250	250	950	130
D	540	90	400	220
E	890	140	1500	280

19. On the basis of the preceding table, the TOTAL number of appointments kept for all clinics in the health center in August is

    A. 900   B. 3910   C. 4810   D. 5710

20. The percentage of appointments kept in Clinic C during August is

    A. 5%   B. 20%   C. 75%   D. 80%

21. If Clinic A was open for 20 days during August, the average number of appointments scheduled each day at Clinic A is

    A. 57   B. 70   C. 140   D. 280

22. In comparison to the clinic which performed the fewest diagnostic procedures, the clinic which performed the MOST diagnostic procedures did _____ as many.

    A. twice   B. three times
    C. four times   D. five times

23. The average number of diagnostic procedures performed for all clinics during August is

    A. 254   B. 676   C. 1352   D. 6760

24. The percentage of all procedures done at Clinic B during August which were surgical procedures is

    A. 2%   B. 2.5%   C. 20%   D. 25%

25. Clinic E used 10 boxes of gauze for its surgical procedures during August. If Clinic A used gauze at the same rate for its surgical procedures, the number of boxes of gauze Clinic A used during August is

    A. 3   B. 5   C. 10   D. 14

KEY (CORRECT ANSWERS)

1. D
2. B
3. A
4. B
5. D

6. C
7. D
8. C
9. B
10. B

11. A
12. C
13. D
14. A
15. C

16. D
17. A
18. C
19. B
20. D

21. B
22. D
23. C
24. C
25. B

TEST 3

DIRECTIONS: Each question or incomplete statement is followed by several suggested answers or completions. Select the one that BEST answers the question or completes the statement. *PRINT THE LETTER OF THE CORRECT ANSWER IN THE SPACE AT THE RIGHT.*

1. Suppose that, in Clinic A, a medical history card is prepared for each new patient. In this clinic, a blood test is made for each patient as a routine procedure. You have been instructed to make out either a blue card for a negative report, or a white card for a positive report, when the laboratory reports of the blood tests are received.
   In order to make sure that all reports on the blood tests have been received, you should compare the number of reports received with the number of

   A. medical history cards
   B. blue cards
   C. white cards
   D. blue cards and white cards

   1.____

2. Assume that there are several clinics within a health center. Patients' cards are filed according to the clinic which they attend, and within each clinic are filed alphabetically. Every Friday you are responsible for filing the cards of all patients who were in the health center during that week. The cards are in mixed order.
   Of the following, the FIRST step to take is to

   A. arrange the patients' cards in alphabetical order
   B. separate the cards of those patients who attended more than one clinic from the others
   C. arrange the patients' cards according to the clinic attended
   D. arrange the patients' cards according to the date the patient attended the clinic

   2.____

3. Assume that the cards of patients are kept in alphabetical order. You are given an alphabetical list of persons who have received injections for *Asian flu* at the clinic and are asked to see if there is a card in the file for each person on the list.
   It would be BEST for you to

   A. determine if the number of cards and the number of names on the list are the same
   B. place a check mark next to each name on the list for which there is a corresponding card
   C. place a check mark on each card for which there is a corresponding name on the list
   D. prepare a second list of all cards in the file and place a check mark next to each name for which there is a corresponding name on the first list

   3.____

4. In filing, a cross index should be used for a record which

   A. may be filed in either of two places
   B. has been temporarily removed from the file
   C. concerns a patient who is no longer coming to the clinic
   D. will be used to remind patients of appointments

   4.____

5. *After washing and rinsing rubber hot water bottles, hang them upside down with their mouths open. When they are thoroughly dry, inflate them, place the stoppers into the mouths of the bottles, and leave them hanging. If they are to be stored, leave them inflated and place gauze or crushed paper between them.*
On the basis of this paragraph, the one of the following statements that is MOST accurate is that, when storing hot water bottles,

   A. they should be stuffed with paper
   B. a free flow of air must circulate around them
   C. care must be taken to prevent their sides from sticking together
   D. they should be placed upside down with their mouths open

6. Assume that when you open a cabinet in which disinfectants are kept, you find that one of the bottles has no label. However, there is a label on the shelf near the bottle.
Of the following, the BEST action for you to take is to

   A. paste the label on the bottle since it obviously is the label for that bottle
   B. paste the label on the bottle only if the label has the word *disinfectant* clearly marked on it
   C. place the bottle back in the cabinet and ask the nurse in charge what to do
   D. pour the contents of the bottle into the sink, rinse the bottle, and place it in the proper receptacle

7. You have been asked to prepare a list of supplies to be reordered for your clinic.
In order for you to determine how much of any item to reorder, it would be MOST important to know

   A. the average amount of the item used in a given period of time
   B. what the item is used for in the clinic
   C. how much storage space is available for these supplies
   D. the cost of each item

8. You have been asked to hand the sterile instruments to the physician while he is changing a dressing. Suppose that halfway through the procedure, the doctor drops the forceps he is using.
Of the following actions, the one that you should take at this time is to

   A. pick up the forceps with your hand and ask the doctor if he will need it any more
   B. pick up the forceps with your hand and place it with other contaminated instruments
   C. move the forceps out of the way with your foot
   D. use sterile forceps from the cabinet to pick up the forceps from the floor

9. If a three-year-old child refuses to stay on a scale long enough to be weighed, the BEST of the following actions for the nurse to take is to

   A. obtain the child's weight by first weighing the mother holding the child in her arms and then weighing the mother alone
   B. insist that the child be weighed so that the other children in the clinic will cooperate when being weighed
   C. ask one of the Special Officers to assist her in weighing the child
   D. note on the record that the child refused to be weighed and let the physician determine if it is necessary to weigh this child

10. Assume that a patient who has been coming to the clinic for some time asks you, *Do I have a heart condition?* You know that his clinic record card bears the notation *heart murmur.*
Under these circumstances, it would be BEST for you to tell him

   A. he has a heart murmur since he obviously knows this and his card gives you the information
   B. he does not have a heart condition since the doctor would have informed the patient if he wanted him to know about it
   C. not to worry about it since lots of people have a heart condition
   D. to ask the physician whom he has been seeing in the clinic about this

11. Suppose that a patient who has just received treatment in the clinic complains loudly that she was kept waiting a long time and then received hasty and inadequate treatment. It is BEST for you to

   A. explain that treatment is necessarily hasty because the clinic is busy
   B. avoid arguing with her since ill people are often overwrought
   C. tell her she is not qualified to decide whether treatment is adequate
   D. refer the patient back to the physician for completion of treatment

12. Assume that you are a nurse assigned to a health center. A middle-aged man walks in and says that he doesn't feel well. He complains of a slight pain in the chest and has difficulty breathing.
Of the following actions, the one you should take is to

   A. isolate him immediately as he may have *Asian flu*
   B. find out what he has eaten as he may have food poisoning
   C. ask him to sit down and see if he can catch his breath
   D. see that he is seated and then call a doctor

13. A baby who has been brought to the health center for an examination has been crying continuously for 20 minutes. The BEST of the following actions you, as a nurse, should take is to

   A. have the baby examined by the first available physician
   B. ask the others who are waiting if they would object to the baby being examined out of turn
   C. call the situation to the attention of the head nurse
   D. do nothing as there are probably others who are ill and need to see the doctor

14. Clinic appointments are LESS likely to be broken if you

   A. make appointments on dates which are convenient for the patients
   B. stress to each patient that a broken appointment inconveniences other patients
   C. threaten not to make any more appointments for patients who break appointments without a good reason
   D. arrange the schedule of appointments so that patients do not have to wait in the clinic

15. Assume that every day the schedule of the clinic is severely disrupted because several patients without appointments must be treated for emergency conditions. Of the following, the BEST suggestion you could make in order to minimize disruption is that

    A. one morning a week be set aside when all emergency cases will be treated
    B. applicants who claim emergency conditions be screened to see which of them really need emergency treatment
    C. unassigned periods be allowed in the schedule in anticipation of emergency cases
    D. the clinic be kept open each evening until all patients have been treated

16. Suppose that a woman who is scheduled to appear at 3:30 PM comes into the clinic at 10 AM and says she is ill and must see the doctor at once. The clinic is already quite crowded.
    It would be BEST for you to

    A. try to determine if she is really ill since some patients use the claim as a ruse to get prompt attention
    B. tell her to return at the proper time since the other patients will become disorderly if others are taken before they are
    C. see if the head nurse will take her out of turn since she may need prompt care
    D. see if a clinic physician is willing to see her since public reaction would be hostile if the condition of the woman became worse while waiting

17. Some authorities advocate that the mother not stay in the same room when a child of 3 or 4 is being treated by the doctor.
    Of the following, the BEST reason for this is that the

    A. mother might become upset if she watches the treatment
    B. child is less likely to accept the doctor's authority
    C. mother will prolong the examination by questioning the doctor about her child
    D. child will mature more rapidly if he is not always accompanied by his mother

18. Assume that a patient tells you that he is not going to follow the treatment recommended by the physician because he doesn't have long to live anyway.
    It would be BEST for you to

    A. report the conversation to the physician
    B. point out to the patient that it is foolish to come for treatment if he will not follow the recommendations given him by the physician
    C. explain to the patient that he will live longer and less painfully if he follows the physician's recommendations
    D. try to get a relative in whom the patient has confidence to persuade him to follow the physician's recommendations

19. Suppose that a mother comes into the health center, where you are a nurse, carrying a 3-year-old child who is ill. The mother tells you that the child has a temperature of 102° F., his nose is stuffed, and he is sneezing.
    For you to seat the mother and child apart from the others who are waiting for the physician is
    A. *correct;* the other children and adults in the clinic should not be exposed to a disease which may be contagious
    B. *incorrect;* the mother might be offended if she were treated differently than the other patients
    C. *correct;* the nurse is in a good position to diagnose patients when the doctor is not available
    D. *incorrect;* you should wait until the physician makes his diagnosis before isolating the child

19._____

20. *In the performance of her work, it is not enough that the nurse be alert to the immediate demands of her own job; she must be constantly aware of the basic function of the clinic.*
    The above statement means that a nurse should view the ultimate purpose of her job as
    A. giving effective service to patients
    B. getting the most work done in the shortest time
    C. following to the letter all orders given to her
    D. reporting punctually and working diligently

20._____

21. As a nurse at an eye clinic, you are instructed to answer the phone by saying, *Eye Clinic, Miss Jones speaking.*
    Of the following, the BEST reason for this practice is that
    A. it sets the tone for a brief, concise telephone conversation
    B. it is the standard practice recommended by the telephone company and is familiar to callers
    C. the caller will understand that he cannot ask for medical information since you are not a physician
    D. the caller will know whether he is speaking to the person he wants to reach

21._____

22. If a telephone call is received for a doctor while he is examining a patient, it would be BEST for the nurse to
    A. tell the caller to telephone again when the doctor can receive a call
    B. take the caller's telephone number and have the doctor return the call when he is free
    C. ask the nature of the call in order to determine if it requires the doctor's immediate attention
    D. refer the call to the nurse in charge as she may have the information the caller requires

22._____

23. Suppose that a patient who attends the clinic has made frequent complaints, usually unjustified.
    Of the following, the BEST reason for not ignoring another complaint from her is that
    A. she is likely to take her complaint to a higher level
    B. even though past complaints have been unjustified, this particular one may require attention
    C. a patient is often pacified if you pretend that you will look into her complaint
    D. no distinction should be made in your attitude toward patients

23._____

24. It is usually recommended that, when new supplies of any item are received, they be placed beneath or behind supplies of the item already in stock.
Of the following, the BEST reason for this is that this procedure

    A. requires less frequent handling of supplies
    B. makes it easier to tell how much of each item you have on hand
    C. allows you to use the storage space most effectively
    D. makes it more likely that the older supplies will be used first

25. Assume that you are in charge of ordering supplies needed for the clinic. When reordering items, it is BEST to

    A. count supplies at the beginning of each month and reorder an item as soon as there is no more of it in stock
    B. determine beforehand the amount of each item which it is necessary to have on hand and reorder the item when the supply falls to this level
    C. reorder each item in sufficient quantity to last half a year so that there will be no danger of running out of supplies
    D. reorder all items at the beginning of each month so that no item needed will be forgotten

---

KEY (CORRECT ANSWERS)

1. A
2. C
3. B
4. A
5. C

6. D
7. A
8. C
9. A
10. D

11. B
12. D
13. C
14. A
15. C

16. C
17. B
18. A
19. A
20. A

21. D
22. C
23. B
24. D
25. B

TEST 4

DIRECTIONS: Each question or incomplete statement is followed by several suggested answers or completions. Select the one that BEST answers the question or completes the statement. *PRINT THE LETTER OF THE CORRECT ANSWER IN THE SPACE AT THE RIGHT.*

1. The drug often used in shock therapy is 1.____
   A. metrazol   B. dicumerol   C. dilantin   D. insulin

2. First aid care of a third degree burn requires 2.____
   A. an ointment
   B. a sterile dressing
   C. opening of the blisters
   D. an antiseptic solution

3. The patient should be kept warm because the blood then 3.____
   A. increases in viscosity
   B. decreases in viscosity
   C. decreases in fluidity
   D. increases in saline content

4. The PRIMARY host for bacteria causing undulant fever is the 4.____
   A. dog   B. goat   C. cow   D. fox

5. Blood clotting is initiated by 5.____
   A. fibrinogen
   B. thromboplastin
   C. calcium ions
   D. vitamin K

6. The MOST accurate way to measure liquid medicine is to use a 6.____
   A. standard teaspoon
   B. standard medicine glass
   C. glass kitchen measuring cup
   D. six-ounce drinking glass

7. In preparing an ice bag, use 7.____
   A. half ice, half water
   B. enough ice to half fill the bag
   C. enough ice to fill the bag
   D. about one pound of ice

8. Morphine 1/4 grain administered 45 minutes before surgery is intended to serve as a 8.____
   A. respiratory depressant
   B. hemotinic
   C. diuretic
   D. hypnotic

9. When putting drops into the eyes of a patient, 9.____
   A. drop them on the eyeball
   B. drop onto the lower lid
   C. use the medication in an eyecup
   D. drop them into the inner corner

10. The safe temperature for water in a hot water bottle for an adult with a normal skin is

    A. 140°-145° F B. 120°-130° F
    C. 100°-125° F D. 110°-115° F

11. The diet in nephritic edema should be

    A. high in vitamins and fluids
    B. low in proteins and fats
    C. high in proteins and minerals
    D. low in fluids and minerals

12. A non-communicable disease is

    A. syphilis   B. pneumonia
    C. carcinoma   D. typhus fever

13. The disease that is transmitted by an insect is

    A. diphtheria   B. typhus fever
    C. scarlet fever D. poliomyelitis

14. Keratitis is an inflammation of the

    A. cornea   B. iris
    C. fundus   D. lachrymal ducts

15. Inflammation of the tear sac is called

    A. dacrocystitis B. cystitis
    C. iritis   D. cyclitis

16. The method now advocated for treating skeletal tuberculosis includes

    A. bed rest and plenty of fresh air
    B. spinal fusion operation
    C. placing patient on a rigid frame
    D. antibiotic therapy, rest, and surgery

17. The nurse rubs the patient's back with alcohol in order to

    A. kill germs on the patient's skin
    B. relax the muscles and prevent bed sores
    C. speed the cure
    D. keep the patient clean

18. When a prescribed medicine is no longer required, it should be

    A. saved for the next illness
    B. disposed of in the garbage or down the drain
    C. given to another patient with a similar illness
    D. administered until all is consumed

19. The purpose of the therapeutic bath is to

    A. cool and refresh B. cleanse
    C. induce sleep   D. improve appearance

20. The PREFERRED method for administering cough medicine is

    A. from the medicine glass
    B. mixed with water
    C. from a spoon
    D. through a siphon tube

21. The hereditary disease in which blood does NOT clot properly is

    A. anemia
    B. leukemia
    C. hemophilia
    D. amoebiosis

22. In first aid a penetrating foreign body in the eyeball should be treated by

    A. removing the object
    B. applying a loose bandage
    C. sending the patient to a doctor
    D. applying a snug bandage

23. A stroke is a(n)

    A. cerebral hemorrhage
    B. sinus thrombosis
    C. cerebral dystrophy
    D. aneurism

24. The aged bed patient is likely to have bed sores because he

    A. is uncooperative
    B. lies in one position and has poor circulation
    C. limits his diet
    D. is uncomfortable

25. Anemia is determined by

    A. color of skin
    B. laboratory techniques
    C. undue fatigue
    D. dizziness without apparent cause

KEY (CORRECT ANSWERS)

1.	D	11.	D
2.	B	12.	C
3.	B	13.	B
4.	B	14.	A
5.	B	15.	A
6.	B	16.	D
7.	B	17.	B
8.	D	18.	B
9.	B	19.	A
10.	B	20.	C

21. C
22. B
23. A
24. B
25. B

TEST 5

DIRECTIONS: Each question or incomplete statement is followed by several suggested answers or completions. Select the one that BEST answers the question or completes the statement. *PRINT THE LETTER OF THE CORRECT ANSWER IN THE SPACE AT THE RIGHT.*

1. Osteomalacia is

    A. a bony tumor
    B. softening of the bones
    C. inflammation of bone marrow
    D. formation of bone

    1.____

2. Asphyxiation may be caused by

    A. heavy concentration of alcohol in the bloodstream
    B. consuming alcohol on an empty stomach
    C. mixing more than one kind of alcoholic drink
    D. taking sedatives while drinking

    2.____

3. An incision of the colon for the purpose of making a fistula is an operation termed

    A. colostration
    B. colostomy
    C. Mikulicz operation
    D. gastrostomy

    3.____

4. Bright's disease is also called

    A. hepatitis
    B. nephritis
    C. Paget's disease
    D. otitis

    4.____

5. Anodyne refers to a medication that

    A. counteracts or removes the effect of poison
    B. relieves pain
    C. prevents the growth of germs
    D. prolongs the life of red blood cells

    5.____

6. Common symptoms of shock are

    A. slow pulse, flushed skin
    B. slow pulse, bright eyes
    C. pale skin, bright eyes
    D. pale, clammy skin

    6.____

7. Adult dietary protein requirements are determined PRIMARILY by

    A. age and weight
    B. climatic conditions
    C. body weight in relation to age and height
    D. muscular activity

    7.____

8. Treatment of generalized arteriosclerosis is through

   A. bed rest
   B. moderation in living
   C. drugs
   D. dealing with the aging process

9. Rugs and carpets should be removed from the sick room because they

   A. collect dust and germs
   B. increase the work in cleaning
   C. produce a static when walked on
   D. present a hazard

10. The administration of narcotics in the hospital is by the

    A. doctor   B. nurse
    C. pharmacist   D. aide

11. Of the following, the factor contributing MOST to apoplexy is

    A. coronary thrombosis   B. aphasia
    C. low blood pressure   D. high blood pressure

12. Croup responds MOST quickly to administrations of

    A. pertussin medication
    B. special diet
    C. steam inhalations
    D. restricted physical movement

13. Euphoria is a state of

    A. depression   B. elation
    C. ideation   D. frustration

14. A drug often used in prevention and treatment of motion sickness is

    A. dramamine   B. streptomycin
    C. atropin   D. aureomycin

15. Of the following, the MOST common cause of death today is

    A. cancer   B. diabetes
    C. heart disease D. pneumonia

16. Cystitis means inflammation of the

    A. kidneys   B. cystic duct
    C. bladder   D. urethra

17. A vesicant is an agent that is used to produce

    A. fever   B. relaxation
    C. lower pulse rate   D. blisters

18. To keep a restless, semi-conscious patient from falling out of bed, we should use 18.____

    A. heavy blankets stretched at the bedside and pinned securely
    B. metal side boards
    C. restraint belts
    D. chairs at the exposed bed side

19. For poisons, swallowed in capsule or tablet form, administer 19.____

    A. a laxative   B. warmth
    C. an emetic   D. a stimulant

20. Oysters which feed on sewage sometimes transmit 20.____

    A. rabies   B. yellow fever
    C. malaria   D. typhoid fever

21. The medium of infection over which the health authorities have LEAST control is 21.____

    A. insects   B. food   C. water   D. air

22. In case of sunstroke, the position of the head is 22.____

    A. lowered, together with the shoulders
    B. elevated, together with the shoulders
    C. bent forward
    D. bent down, between the knees

23. Encephalitis has NOT been associated with 23.____

    A. infectious illnesses   B. epidemics
    C. measles   D. drugs

24. The Sulkowitch test of the urine tests for 24.____

    A. sodium   B. potassium
    C. calcium   D. chlorides

25. The presence of acetone in urine indicates faulty metabolism of 25.____

    A. proteins   B. fats
    C. carbohydrates   D. minerals

KEY (CORRECT ANSWERS)

1. B
2. A
3. B
4. B
5. B

6. D
7. C
8. B
9. D
10. B

11. D
12. C
13. B
14. A
15. C

16. C
17. D
18. B
19. C
20. D

21. D
22. B
23. D
24. C
25. C

TEST 6

DIRECTIONS: Each question or incomplete statement is followed by several suggested answers or completions. Select the one that BEST answers the question or completes the statement. *PRINT THE LETTER OF THE CORRECT ANSWER IN THE SPACE AT THE RIGHT.*

1. The test which aids the physician in confirming infectious mononucleosis is

    A. urinalysis
    B. Wasserman
    C. sedementation rate
    D. heterophile antibody test

2. The purpose of the therapeutic bath is to

    A. cool and refresh
    B. cleanse
    C. induce sleep
    D. improve appearance

3. Syphilis is transmitted to the fetus through the

    A. ovum
    B. embryonic fluid
    C. placenta
    D. sperm

4. A nurse can be of GREATEST help to the doctor by

    A. applying mental hygiene procedures
    B. suggesting treatments
    C. recording observations accurately
    D. minimizing the patients' complaints

5. BCG vaccine is used to increase resistance to

    A. poliomyelitis
    B. tuberculosis
    C. smallpox
    D. mumps

6. In order to prevent rickets, the diet should include

    A. carotene   B. calciferol   C. riboflavin   D. thiamin

7. To a dog bite wound apply

    A. 2% iodine
    B. concentrated boric acid
    C. carbolated vaseline
    D. running water

8. To prevent constipation in the aged, we should use

    A. enemas
    B. phenolthaleine
    C. mineral oil
    D. proper diet

9. Seafood should be included in the diet at least once a week because of

    A. religion
    B. its iodine content
    C. its iron content
    D. variety appeal

10. For the patient, the MOST comfortable mattress protection is a

    A. rubber draw sheet
    B. plastic pad
    C. quilted pad
    D. plastic contour *sheet*

11. To relieve the sensitive-skinned patient from bed pressure, use a(n)

    A. inflated mattress B. inflated rubber ring
    C. cotton bandage ring D. sponge rubber ring

12. A symptom of diabetes is

    A. oliguria B. polyuria C. anuria D. hematuria

13. The disease characterized by the abnormal mitosis and development of body cells is

    A. influenza B. Parkinson's disease
    C. carcinoma D. Graves' disease

14. The water used in preparing a mustard plaster should be

    A. boiling B. cold C. tepid D. hot

15. To stimulate peristalsis, the fluid in colonic irrigations should be

    A. cool B. lukewarm C. warm D. hot

16. In ear irrigation, the external ear is straightened by pulling the pinna

    A. down and back B. down and forward
    C. up and forward D. up and back

17. Hypoglycemia indicates the need for the administration of

    A. adrenalin B. a simple sugar
    C. insulin D. salt

18. To reduce swelling, apply

    A. hot applications B. cold applications
    C. electric heating pad D. a snug bandage

19. The value of antihistaminic compounds lies PRIMARILY in their ability to

    A. prevent the spread of infection
    B. relieve the allergic manifestations
    C. lessen the number of infections
    D. immunize

20. Very hot and very cold foods, fed to a patient with acute myocardial infarction, can cause irregular heart beat by irritating the _____ nerve.

    A. median B. common peronal
    C. deep peronal D. vagus

21. Tachycardia is also known as

    A. high blood pressure B. low blood pressure
    C. rapid pulse D. slow pulse

22. Dyspnea is

    A. blurring vision B. pain around the heart
    C. difficult breathing D. discoloration of the skin

23. Manifest deviation of one eye when looking at an object is called

 A. strabismus B. astigmatism
 C. accommodation D. glaucoma

24. Abnormally slow pulse is referred to as

 A. tachycardia B. intermittent
 C. arrhythmia D. bradycardia

25. Dilatin is a medication used in the treatment of

 A. cardiac involvement B. multiple sclerosis
 C. grand mal D. cerebral palsy

KEY (CORRECT ANSWERS)

1. D   11. A
2. A   12. B
3. C   13. C
4. C   14. C
5. B   15. A

6. B   16. D
7. D   17. B
8. D   18. B
9. B   19. B
10. C   20. D

21. C
22. C
23. A
24. D
25. C

TEST 7

DIRECTIONS: Each question or incomplete statement is followed by several suggested answers or completions. Select the one that BEST answers the question or completes the statement. *PRINT THE LETTER OF THE CORRECT ANSWER IN THE SPACE AT THE RIGHT.*

1. The MOST practical bed sheet is made of

    A. muslin
    B. broadcloth
    C. nylon
    D. linen

2. Decubitus is another name for

    A. mental derangement
    B. dyspnea
    C. decayed teeth
    D. bedsore

3. Of the following, the non-infectious disease is

    A. hepatitis
    B. poliomyelitis
    C. diabetes
    D. impetigo

4. The CHIEF purpose of isolating a patient is to

    A. protect others
    B. prevent reinfection
    C. hasten recovery
    D. provide peace and comfort

5. In giving first aid treatment to a person who has fainted,

    A. administer a hot beverage
    B. hold the head back and open the mouth
    C. administer aromatic spirits of ammonia
    D. lower the head below heart level

6. A drug which is a substitute for morphine in the treatment of drug addiction is

    A. codeine   B. demerol   C. pantapon   D. methadone

7. The drug having LEAST narcotic effect per unit of weight is

    A. marijuana
    B. cocaine
    C. opium
    D. barbiturates

8. An hypnotic drug which does NOT initiate drug addiction is

    A. dormison
    B. sodium amytal
    C. sodium phenobarbital
    D. seconal

9. A term meaning *farsightedness* is

    A. hyperopia
    B. nystagmus
    C. strabismus
    D. myopia

10. Cholecystography is the x-ray examination of the

    A. stomach
    B. spleen
    C. gall bladder
    D. intestines

11. Pyelonephritis is an inflammation of the

   A. kidney   B. pancreas   C. rectum   D. mastoid

12. Pellagra results from a deficiency of

   A. ascorbic acid   B. thiamine
   C. riboflavin   D. niacin

13. Cheilosis results from a deficiency of

   A. pyrodoxin   B. vitamin E
   C. riboflavin   D. niacin

14. Folic acid, used in the treatment of pernicious anemia, must be given with vitamin

   A. B_1 B. B_2 C. B_6 D. B_{12}

15. Radioactive iodine compound is fed to determine the

   A. site of red blood cell production
   B. incidence of anemia
   C. presence of cholesterol
   D. thyroid activity

16. Predisposition to epilepsy may be discovered through the use of

   A. stethoscope   B. fluoroscope
   C. encephalograph   D. opthalmoscope

17. An early symptom of glaucoma is

   A. blindness
   B. gradual loss of side vision
   C. excessive tearing
   D. cataract formation

18. A kind of nervous headache usually periodical and confined to one side of the head is

   A. pressure   B. vertigo   C. migraine   D. traumatic

19. Rocky Mountain spotted fever is spread by

   A. rodents
   B. ticks
   C. sewage disposal in rivers
   D. contaminated water supply

20. The Rh factor must be considered carefully when giving a(n)

   A. restricted diet   B. intravenous medication
   C. antibiotic medication   D. transfusion

21. The CHIEF action of ACTH is to

   A. relieve arthritic pain and swelling
   B. cure arthritis
   C. stimulate production of cortisone
   D. extend benefits gained in surgical procedures

22. Vitamin K has NO effect on hemorrhage

   A. in infants
   B. in surgery
   C. due to hemophilia
   D. associated with obstructive jaundice

23. Opthalmia neontorum is the medical term meaning

   A. eye infection of infants
   B. blindness
   C. cross-eyedness
   D. astigmatism

24. A non-catagious disease caused by a soil fungus is

   A. histoplasmosis   B. xeropthalmia
   C. jaundice   D. keratitis

25. Vaccination against Rocky Mountain spotted fever must be given

   A. every seven years   B. promptly upon infection
   C. every year   D. in rat-infested areas

KEY (CORRECT ANSWERS)

1.	A	11.	A
2.	D	12.	D
3.	C	13.	A
4.	A	14.	D
5.	D	15.	D
6.	D	16.	C
7.	A	17.	B
8.	A	18.	C
9.	A	19.	B
10.	C	20.	D

21. B
22. C
23. A
24. A
25. A

EXAMINATION SECTION
TEST 1

DIRECTIONS: Each question or incomplete statement is followed by several suggested answers or completions. Select the one that BEST answers the question or completes the statement. *PRINT THE LETTER OF THE CORRECT ANSWER IN THE SPACE AT THE RIGHT*

Questions 1-10.

DIRECTIONS: Questions 1 through 10 are to be answered on the basis of the following information.

58-year-old Julie Fields is brought to the hospital by her husband after having enlarged nodes in the lower cervical region. Mrs. Fields also has fever and complains of night sweats.

1. After being examined by the physician, Mrs. Fields is diagnosed with Hodgkin's lymphoma, which may BEST be described as a(n) _____ disease with _____ that may be present in localized or disseminated form.
    A. chronic; lymphatic proliferation
    B. acute; reticular proliferation
    C. chronic; lymphoreticular proliferation of unknown cause
    D. acute; lymphoreticular proliferation of various causes

1._____

2. Which of the following is NOT a true fact about the incidence of Hodgkin's lymphoma?
    A. Annually in the United States, 5000 to 6000 new cases are diagnosed.
    B. The male: female ratio is 1.4:1.
    C. Rare before age 10, a binodal age distribution exists with one peak at ages 15 to 34 and another after age 54.
    D. Epidemiologic studies find considerable evidence of horizontal spread.

2._____

3. A CORRECT etiology finding about Hodgkin's lymphoma is:
    A. It resembles a low-grade graft-versus-host reaction
    B. Recent. evidence of tumor-associated antigens in Hodgkin's tissue is consistent with interpretation given in para A
    C. A number of infectious agents, including viruses, are postulated as causes
    D. All of the above

3._____

4. The one of the following that is NOT one of the four histopathologic classifications of Hodgkin's lymphoma is:
    A. Lymphocyte predominance - few Reed-Sternberg cells and many lymphocytes
    B. Mixed cellularity - an increased number of Reed-Sternberg cells with a mixed infiltrate
    C. Nodular sclerosis - generally, a moderate number of Reed-Sternberg cells with a mixed infiltrate except that dense fibrous tissue, which shows characteristic birefringence with polarized light, surrounds nodules of Hodgkin's tissue
    D. Lymphocyte depletion - few lymphocytes, numerous Reed-Sternberg cells, and extensive fibrosis or abnormal reticulum cell infiltrate

4._____

5. While assessing Mrs. Fields, the nurse may expect to notice all of the following EXCEPT
    A. pruritis and petechiae
    B. recurrent, intermittent fever
    C. weight loss, malaise, and lethargy
    D. enlarged nodes in the lower cervical region; nodes are nontender, firm, and moveable

5._____

6. The diagnosis of Hodgkin's lymphoma depends upon the identification of
   A. small multinucleated lymphatic cells in lymph node tissue
   B. large multinucleated reticulum cells, also named Reed-Sternberg cells, in lymph node tissue or other sites
   C. large multinucleated lymphoreticular cells in lymph nodes
   D. all of the above

7. Which of the following will NOT be part of Mrs. Fields' medical management?
   A. Lymphangiogram: determines the involvement of all the lymph nodes, is reliable in 90% of patients, and is helpful in determining radiation fields
   B. Laparotomy and splenectomy
   C. Lymph node biopsy to identify the presence of Reed-Sternberg cells and for hematologic classification
   D. Radiation: used alone for localized disease

8. Hodgkin's lymphoma staging via laparotomy and biopsy shows all of the following except Stage
   A. I: single lymph node involved, usually in neck, 90% to 98% survival
   B. II: involvement of 6 or more lymph nodes on same side of diaphragm, 70-80% survival
   C. III: involvement of lymph nodes on both sides of diaphragm, 50% survival
   D. IV: metastasis to other organs

9. Chemotherapy is used in conjunction with radiation therapy for advanced disease. The drug combination of choice for Hodgkin's lymphoma is
   A. adriamycin, bleomycin, procarbazine, and prednisone (ABPP)
   B. mechlorethamine vincristine (oncovin), adriamycin, and dacarbazine (MOAD)
   C. nitrosoureas, streptozocin, cis-platinum, and epipodophyllotoxin (VP-16)
   D. mechlorethamine, vincristine (oncovin), procarbazine, and prednisone (MOPP)

10. An IMPORTANT nursing intervention for Hodgkin's lymphoma would be to
    A. provide care for a patient receiving radiation therapy
    B. administer chemotherapy as ordered and monitor/ alleviate the side effects
    C. protect patients from infection, especially if splenectomy is performed
    D. all of the above

Questions 11-18.

DIRECTIONS: Questions 11 through 18 are to be answered on the basis of the following information.
   36-year-old Nancy Drew is brought to the hospital by her husband after having marked respiratory distress. Mrs. Drew also has a family history of allergies.

11. After being examined, Mrs. Drew is diagnosed with bronchial asthma, which may be accurately described by all of the following EXCEPT:
    A. A reversible obstructive lung disorder characterized by increased responsiveness of the airways
    B. Often caused by an allergic reaction to an environmental allergen, and always Seasonal
    C. Immunologic/allergic reaction results in histamine release, which produces three main airway responses, i.e., edema of mucous membranes and spasm of the smooth muscle of bronchi and bronchioles and accumulation of tenacious secretions
    D. Status asthmaticus occurs when there is little response to treatment and symptoms persist

12. The one of the following pathophysiological findings that is NOT true about bronchial asthma is:
    A. Airway obstruction causes hypoventilation in some lung areas, and continued blood flow to these areas leads to a ventilation/perfusion imbalance resulting in hypoxemia. Arterial hypoxemia is almost always present in attacks severe enough to require medical attention.
    B. Hyperventilation occurs early in the attack and results in a decrease in $PaCO_2$. As the attack progresses, the patient's capacity to compensate by hyperventilation of unobstructed areas of the lung is further impaired by more extensive airways narrowing and muscular fatigue. Arterial hypoxemia worsens and $PaCO_2$ begins to rise, leading respiratory acidosis. At this point, the patient is said to be in respiratory failure, stage IV of an acute attack.
    C. An imbalance between 13-adrenergic and cholinergic control of airways diameter has been proposed, one of the facts being a decreased cholinergic responsiveness because most asthmatics respond excessively with bronchoconstriction after inhalation of cholinergic agents and because atropine and its derivatives can often partially block irritant-induced bronchocon-striction.
    D. The observed abnormalities in adrenergic and cholinergic functions in asthma appear to be controlled by the cyclic 31,51 - adenosine monophosphate (Camp) cyclic 3',5' - guanosine monophosphate (cGMP) systems within various tissues, e.g., mast cells, smooth muscle, and mucus-secreting cells

13. While assessing Mrs. Drew, the nurse may expect to notice all of the following EXCEPT
    A. family history of infections by gram-negative aerobic cocci
    B. patient history of eczema
    C. shortness of breath, expiratory wheeze, prolonged expiratory phase, air trapping (barrel chest if chronic)
    D. use of accessory muscles, irritability (from hypoxia), diaphoresis, change in sensorium if severe attack

14. Which of the following is NOT true regarding laboratory finding in asthma?
    A. Eosinophilia is commonly present, regardless of whether allergic factors can be shown to have an etiologic role. Blood eosinophilia greater than 250 to 400 cells/µL is the rule.
    B. Determination of arterial blood gases and pH is essential to the adequate evaluation of a patient with asthma of sufficient severity to warrant hospitalization.
    C. Chest x-ray findings varying from normal to hypo-inflation. Lung markings are increased, particularly in chronic disease. The expiratory x-rays are especially important in the case of non-opaque foreign bodies.
    D. Pulmonary function tests are valuable in differential diagnosis, and also in known asthmatics to assess the degree of airway obstruction and disturbance in gas exchange, to measure the airways' response to inhaled allergens and chemicals, to quantify the response to drugs, and for long-term follow-up

15. The INCORRECT statement about diagnostic tests for asthma is
    A. Static lung volumes and capacities reveal various combinations of abnormalities. Of the tests most often used clinically, total lung capacity (TLC), functional residual capacity (FRC), and residual volume (RV) are usually increased. Vital capacity (VC) may be normal or increased.
    B. The confirmation of extrinsic allergic factors is best accomplished by an allergy evaluation that includes allergy skin testing with extracts to detect IgE antibody to inhalants and other allergens suggested by the patient's history.

C. Specific IgE antibody to inhalants may also be detected by a radioallergosorbent test (RAST) on the patient's serum, but this test is expensive, subject to laboratory error, and offers little advantage over properly done and interpreted skin tests.
D. Inhalational bronchial challenge testing has been used (1) with allergens to establish the clinical significance of positive skin tests, (2) with methacoline or histamine to assess the degree of airway hyperactivity in known asthmatics, or (3) to aid in diagnosing asthma when the symptoms are atypical.

16. When performing a physical examination of a patient with asthma, the one of the following that does NOT apply is:
    A. You should search for heart failure and signs of chronic hypoxemia, such as clubbing of the fingers
    B. Nasal polyposis should suggest aspirin intolerance
    C. A unilateral wheezing should provoke a search for obstruction by a foreign body, vascular malformation, aneurysm, or tumor
    D. In tracheal obstruction, an inspiratory wheeze is present over the lower airway

17. All of the following would be appropriate nursing interventions to control Mrs. Drew's condition EXCEPT:
    A. administering oxygen as ordered and placing patient in low-Fowler's position
    B. providing humidification/hydration to loosen secretions
    C. providing chest percussion and postural drainage when bronchodilation improves
    D. monitoring for respiratory distress

18. Mrs. Drew has recovered and is ready to be discharged.
    The nurse will provide her with teaching and discharge planning concerning all of the following EXCEPT
    A. stay indoors during grass cutting or when pollen count is high
    B. avoid natural fibers like wool and feathers; avoid rugs, stuffed animals, and draperies or curtains
    C. importance of moderate exercises with contraindication of swimming
    D. purpose of breathing exercises to increase the end expiratory pressure of each respiration

Questions 19-26.

DIRECTIONS: Questions 19 through 26 are to be answered on the basis of the following information.
48-year-old Moe Link is admitted into the hospital because of mild chest pain. He is 5 feet, 8 inches tall and weighs 198 pounds. A myocardial infarction is diagnosed.

19. Oxygen by nasal cannula is prescribed for Mr. Link. Safety precautions would be used by the nurse in the room because oxygen
    A. has unstable properties
    B. may convert to an alternate form
    C. is flammable
    D. supports combustion

20. Isoenzyme laboratory studies are ordered.
    The isoenzyme test that is the MOST reliable early indicator of myocardial insult is
    A. AST   B. SGPT   C. CPK   D. LDH

21. An electrocardiogram is ordered. 21._____
    An early finding in the lead over the infarcted area would be
    A. absence of T waves   B. flattened P waves
    C. elevated ST segments   D. disappearance of Q waves

22. The physician orders 8 mg. of morphine sulfate to be given by injection. The vial on hand   22._____
    is labeled 1 ml =10 mg.
    The nurse should administer _____ minims.
    A. 8   B. 12   C. 16   D. 20

23. Mr. Link wants to know why he is given the injection of morphine.   23._____
    The nurse explains to him that it
    A. decreases anxiety and restlessness
    B. contracts coronary b000d vessels
    C. relieves pain and prevents shock
    D. helps prevent fibrillation of heart

24. Mr. Link, who was admitted three days earlier, is complaining to the nurse about   24._____
    numerous aspects of his hospital stay.
    The BEST initial nursing response would be to
    A. try to explain the purpose of different hospital routines
    B. refocus the conversation on his anger, fears, and frustrations about his condition
    C. allow him to express his feelings and then promptly leave to permit him to regain his composure
    D. explain how his upset condition dangerously interferes with his need for rest

25. Several days after admission, Mr. Link develops pyrexia.   25._____
    One of the adaptations related to the pyrexia that the nurse would monitor him for
    would be
    A. depressed blood pressure
    B. back pain
    C. increased pulse rate
    D. dyspnea

26. Mr. Link asks the nurse about his chances of having another heart attack if he watches   26._____
    his diet and stress levels carefully.
    The MOST appropriate initial response by the nurse would be to
    A. avoid giving him direct information and help him explore his feelings
    B. suggest to him that he discuss his feelings of vulnerability with his physician
    C. recognize that he is frightened and suggest that he talk with the psychologic nurse
    D. tell him that he certainly needs to be careful in these areas

Questions 27-30.
DIRECTIONS: Questions 27 through 30 are to be answered on the basis of the following information.
56-year-old Holly Parton is having a workup for pernicious anemia.

27. A Schilling test is ordered for Mrs. Parton.   27._____
    The nurse should know that the PRIMARY purpose of the Schilling test is to determine
    the patient's ability to _____ vitamin B_{12}.
    A. produce   B. metabolize   C. store   D. absorb

28. Pernicious anemia is confirmed, and the physician orders 0.4 mg of cyanocobalamin IM. The available vial of the drug is labeled 1 ml = 100 mcg. The nurse should administer _____ ml.
    A. 1   B. 2   C. 3   D. 4

29. When you tell Mrs. Parton the therapeutic regimen about vitamin B12, the nurse should tell her that
    A. intramuscular injections are required weekly for control
    B. oral supplements taken daily will control her symptoms
    C. intramuscular injections once a month will control the symptoms
    D. monthly Z-track injections will provide the required control

30. Mrs. Parton understands the instructions regarding the vitamin B_{12} injections when the nurse states that she must take it
    A. during exacerbations of anemia
    B. when she feels hypertensed
    C. until her symptoms are controlled
    D. for the rest of her life

KEY (CORRECT ANSWERS)

1. C	11. B	21. C
2. D	12. C	22. B
3. D	13. A	23. C
4. B	14. C	24. B
5. A	15. A	25. C
6. B	16. D	26. A
7. C	17. A	27. D
8. B	18. C	28. D
9. D	19. D	29. C
10. D	20. C	30. D

TEST 2

DIRECTIONS: Each question or incomplete statement is followed by several suggested answers or completions. Select the one that BEST answers the question or completes the statement. *PRINT THE LETTER OF THE CORRECT ANSWER IN THE SPACE AT THE RIGHT*

Questions 1-12.
DIRECTIONS: Questions 1 through 12 are to be answered on the basis of the following information.

46-year-old Tanya Hardin is brought to the hospital by her husband after having enlarged lymph nodes which are rubbery and discrete. Mrs. Hardin also complains of weight loss and fever with night sweats.

1. After being examined by the physician, Mrs. Hardin is diagnosed with Non-Hodgkin's lymphoma, which may BEST be described as
   A. a heterogeneous group of diseases consisting of neo-plastic proliferation of lymphoid cells that usually disseminate throughout the body
   B. a heterogeneous group of diseases, which includes a wide range of disease entities, e.g., lymphosarcoma, reticulum cell sarcoma, and Burkitt's lymphoma
   C. primary sites include gastrointestinal tract, ovaries, testes, bones, CNS, liver, breast, and subcutaneous tissues
   D. all of the above

1.____

2. Which of the following age groups is MOST affected by Non-Hodgkin's lymphoma?
   A. Women age 40 and over
   B. Men age 40 and over
   C. Both men and women age 40 and over
   D. All age groups

2.____

3. Close association of Type _____ with some adult leukemias and lymphomas comprised of peripheral T cells has been demonstrated in recent years.
   A. adenovirus   B. rhinovirus   C. retrovirus   D. reovirus

3.____

4. Of the following human T-cell leukemia-lymphoma viruses (HTLV), the one that has been isolated from several patients and appears to be endemic to Japan, the Caribbean, South America, and certain regions of the United States is HTLV-
   A. I   B. II   C. III   D. IV

4.____

5. The Rappaport classification for the histopathology of NHL is based on the degree of differentiation of the tumor, and on the presence or absence of nodules. All classes are divided into nodular or diffuse.
   The class that occurs ONLY in a diffuse pattern is malignant lymphoma,
   A. histiocytic
   B. undifferentiated Burkitt's type or non-Burkitt's pleomorphic type
   C. lymphocytic
   D. mixed lymphocytic-histiocytic

5.____

35

6. The Lukes and Collins classification, which is based upon the cell of origin, divides NHL into
   A. T cell (thymus-derived) types that include immunoblastic sarcoma and convoluted cell lymphoma, similar to lymphoblastic lymphoma. Occurs in about 15% of all cases.
   B. cell (bone marrow-derived) types that include well-differentiated lymphocytic, plasmacytic, follicular center cell lymphomas, and a B-cell immunoblastic sarcoma. Occurs in about 75% of all cases.
   C. true histiocytic or monocytic origin type. Occurs in about 5% of all cases.
   D. all of the above

7. The new International Panel Working Formulation separates NHL into all of the following categories EXCEPT _____, described as _____ types.
   A. *low grade or favorable-prognosis lymphomas*; diffuse, well-differentiated; nodular, poorly differentiated lymphocytic; and nodular-mixed
   B. *intermediate-grade or prognosis lymphomas*; nodular histiocytic; diffuse, poorly differentiated, lymphocytic; and diffuse-mixed
   C. *high grade or unfavorable-prognosis lymphomas*; diffuse histiocytic lymphoma; diffuse undifferentiated; and lymphoblastic T cell lymphoma
   D. *highest grade or no prognosis lymphomas*; non-composite lymphomas, false histiocytic, other, and unclassifiable

8. While assessing Mrs. Hardin, the nurse should NOT expect to notice
   A. asymptomatic adenopathy involving cervical or inguinal regions, or both
   B. anemia, which is initially present in about 33% of patients and eventually develops in most. It may be due to bleeding from GI involvement or low platelet levels, hemolysis due to hypersplenism or Coombs-positive hemolytic anemia, bone marrow infiltration by lymphoma, or marrow suppression by drugs or irradiation
   C. a leukemic phase, which develops in 40-60% of lymphocytic lymphomas and 20% of histiocytic lymphomas
   D. hypogammaglobulinemia due to progressive decrease in immunoglobulin production, which occurs in 15% of patients and may predispose to serious bacterial infection

9. All of the following are correct about the treatment of early NHL disease (stages I and II) EXCEPT:
   A. With low and intermediate-grade lymphomas, patients rarely present with localized disease, but, when they do, regional radiotherapy offers long-term control and sometimes cure
   B. Those with high-grade lymphomas are generally treated with combination chemotherapy with or without regional radiotherapy
   C. Cure rates vary from 40 to 60%
   D. None of the above

10. In the treatment of advanced disease (stages III and IV),
    A. a watch and wait approach, treatment with a single alkylating agent, or 2- and 3-drug programs may be used
    B. interferon as well as other biologic response modifiers have resulted in some encouraging remissions
    C. while survival may be prolonged, relapse eventually occurs and cure rates are generally less than 20 to 25%
    D. all of the above

11. In patients with intermediate-grade lymphomas, combinations of certain drugs with or without adriamycin result in complete regression of disease in 50 to 70% of patients. In these cases, a pattern of continuous late relapse usually occurs, however, and only 20 to 30% are cured.
    These drugs are _____, vincristine, and _____.
    A. procarbazine; prednisone
    B. cyclophosphamide; prednisone
    C. mechlorethamine; procarbazine
    D. nitrosoureas; streptozocin

    11._____

12. Patients having lymphomas with unfavorable-prognosis histology usually have rapid tumor growth (high grade), but modern intensive combination chemotherapy programs have dramatically reversed the previously poor cure rate of less than 10%.
    Use of a _____ drug program with acronyms has resulted in complete remission rates of 50 to 70% with about 40 to 60% of all patients being cured.
    A. 4   B. 5   C. 6   D. all of the above

    12._____

Questions 13-20.

DIRECTIONS: Questions 13 through 20 are to be answered on the basis of the following information.
56-year-old Jerry West visits the hospital after having a cough with sputum production, anorexia, and fatigue. Mr. West has also been a cigarette smoker since he was 20.

13. After being examined by the physician, Mr. West is diagnosed with emphysema. All of the following statements give correct information about the disease EXCEPT:
    A. Contraction of tracheal muscles with resultant loss of recoil occurs
    B. Enlargement and destruction of the alveolar, bronchial, and bronchiolar tissue with resultant loss of recoil, air trapping, thoracic overdistension, sputum accumulation, and loss of diaphragmatic muscle tone occur
    C. The changes given above in B. cause a state of carbon dioxide retention, hypoxia, and respiratory acidosis
    D. The disease is caused by cigarette smoking, infection, inhaled irritants, heredity, allergic factors, and aging

    13._____

14. While assessing Mr. West, the nurse will NOT expect to notice
    A. weight loss and decreased rate and depth of breathing
    B. dyspnea, feeling of breathlessness, and sputum production
    C. flaring of the nostrils and use of accessory muscles of respiration
    D. decreased respiratory excursion, resonance to hyper-resonance, decreased breath sounds with prolonged expiration, and normal or decreased fremitus

    14._____

15. A CORRECT diagnostic test finding for emphysema is PCO_2 _____ and PO_2 _____.
    A. elevated; normal
    B. normal; slightly decreased
    C. elevated; slightly increased
    D. elevated or normal; normal or slightly decreased

    15._____

16. All of the following are accurate pathological findings of emphysema EXCEPT:
    A. Microscopic examination reveals departitioning of the lung due to loss of alveolar walls; large bullae may be present in advanced disease
    B. In severe emphysema, the lungs are large and pale and always fail to collapse when the thorax is opened
    C. Changes may be most marked in the center of the acinus, i.e., centrilobular emphysema or more diffusely scattered throughout the lobule, i.e., panacinar emphysema. In all forms, normal architecture is destroyed and loss of alveolar walls results in air sacs of various sizes.
    D. The abnormalities lead not only to a reduction in the area of alveolar membrane available for gas exchange, but also to the perfusion of nonventilated areas and to the ventilation of nonperfused parts of the lung, i.e., ventilation/perfusion (V/Q) abnormalities

17. CORRECT drug therapy in the treatment of emphysema includes the use of
    A. bronchodilators such as aminophylline, isoproterenol (isuprel), terbutaline (brethine), metaproterenol (alupent), theophylline, and isoetharine (bronkosol) to treat bronchospasm
    B. tetracycline and ampicillin to treat bacterial infections
    C. prednisone as a corticosteroid
    D. all of the above

18. All of the following would be appropriate nursing interventions to control Mr. West's condition EXCEPT
    A. assuring fluid intake of at least 5 liters a day
    B. facilitating removal of secretions by providing chest physical therapy, coughing, and deep breathing, and use of hand nebulizers
    C. improving ventilation by placing him in semi- or high-Fowler's position
    D. instructing him to use diaphragmatic muscle to breathe; employing pursed-lip breathing techniques

19. All of the following would be appropriate teaching and discharge planning provided by the nurse to Mr. West concerning prevention of recurrent infections EXCEPT;
    A. Avoid crowds and individuals with known infection
    B. Adhere to a high-protein, high-carbohydrate, and increased vitamin C diet
    C. Receive immunizations for influenza, pneumonia, and tuberculosis
    D. Report changes in characteristics and color of sputum immediately; report Worsening of symptoms like increased tightness of chest, fatigue, and increased dyspnea

20. Which of the following will NOT be a part of teaching and discharge planning provided by the nurse to Mr. West concerning environmental control and avoidance of inhaled irritants?
    A. Use home humidifier at 30-50% humidity
    B. Wear a scarf over nose and mouth in very hot weather to prevent bronchospasm
    C. Avoid smoking and others who smoke; avoid abrupt changes in temperature
    D. Use an air conditioner with a high-efficiency particulate air filter to remove particles from the air

Questions 21-25.

DIRECTIONS: Questions 21 through 25 are to be answered on the basis of the following information.

22-year-old David Quinn, a military recruit, visits the hospital after having a fever and enlarged, red tonsils.

21. After being examined by the physician, David is diagnosed with tonsillitis, which is a (n) _____, usually due to _____ infection.
    A. acute inflammation of the tonsils; streptococcal or, less commonly, fungal
    B. chronic inflammation of the tonsils; bacterial or, less commonly, viral
    C. acute inflammation of the palatine tonsils; streptococcal or, less commonly, viral
    D. chronic inflammation of the palatine tonsils; staphylococcal or, less commonly, streptococcal

21._____

22. _____% of tonsillitis is caused by group A beta-hemolytic streptococci.
    A. 10-15   B. 15-20   C. 20-25   D. 25-30

22._____

23. While assessing David, the nurse may expect to notice all of the following EXCEPT
    A. sore throat and pain, most marked on swallowing and often referred to the nostrils
    B. high fever, malaise, headache, and vomiting
    C. white patches of exudate on tonsillar pillars
    D. enlarged cervical lymph nodes

23._____

24. Penicillin G or V is the treatment of choice for streptococcal tonsillitis and should be continued for 10 days.
    The APPROPRIATE dosage would be _____ every _____ hours.
    A. 250 mg orally; 6   B. 325 mg IM; 8   C. 500 mg IV; 10   D. all of the above

24._____

25. When possible, the patient's throat should be recultured 5 to 6 days after treatment is over. Family members' throats should also be cultured initially so that carriers may be treated at the same time.
    Tonsillectomy should be considered if
    A. despite the above given precautions acute tonsillitis repeatedly develops after adequate treatment
    B. chronic tonsillitis and sore throat persist
    C. chronic tonsillitis and sore throat are relieved only briefly by antibiotic therapy
    D. all of the above

25._____

KEY (CORRECT ANSWERS)

1.	D	11.	B
2.	D	12.	D
3.	C	13.	A
4.	A	14.	A
5.	B	15.	D
6.	D	16.	B
7.	D	17.	D
8.	C	18.	A
9.	D	19.	C
10.	D	20.	B

21. C
22. A
23. A
24. A
25. D

EXAMINATION SECTION
TEST 1

DIRECTIONS: Each question or incomplete statement is followed by several suggested answers or completions. Select the one that BEST answers the question or completes the statement. *PRINT THE LETTER OF THE CORRECT ANSWER IN THE SPACE AT THE RIGHT.*

Questions 1-10.

DIRECTIONS: Questions 1 through 10 are to be answered on the basis of the following information.

Newly delivered, 34-year-old Susan Robinson comes to the hospital after feeling pain and noticing swollen, dilated, and tortuous skin veins in her lower extremities.

1. The physican examines Mrs. Robinson and makes a diagnosis of varicose veins, which is BEST described as elongated, dilated, tortuous superficial veins whose valves _____ , the condition occurring most often in the _____.

    A. are congenitally absent; lower extremities
    B. are scant; upper extremities
    C. have become incompetent; trunk
    D. are congenitally absent, scant, or have become incompetent; lower extremities and trunk

1.____

2. Varicose veins are MOST commonly found in _____ ages _____.

    A. women; 40 to 60
    B. men; 40 to 60
    C. women; 30 to 50
    D. both men and women; 30 to 50

2.____

3. All of the following are known to be predisposing factors for varicose veins EXCEPT

    A. congenital weakness of the veins
    B. obesity
    C. liver disease
    D. pregnancy

3.____

4. While assessing Mrs. Robinson, the nurse will NOT expect to notice

    A. pain after prolonged standing
    B. pain relieved by elevation
    C. tortuous skin veins
    D. deep, swollen and dilated veins

4.____

5. Which of the following would be used as a diagnostic test for Mrs. Robinson?

    A. X-rays
    B. Venography
    C. Plethysmography
    D. The Trendelenburg test

5.____

41

6. The one of the following that is NOT considered among the treatments for varicose veins is

   A. venography
   B. vein ligation
   C. injection sclerotherapy
   D. lightweight compression hosiery for small, mildly symptomatic varicose veins

7. All of the following would be appropriate nursing interventions for Mrs. Robinson EXCEPT

   A. measuring the circumference of the ankle and calf at least every 8 hours
   B. elevating legs above heart level
   C. applying knee-length elastic stockings
   D. providing adequate rest

8. It would NOT be an appropriate nursing intervention for vein ligation to

   A. keep the affected extremity above the level of the heart to prevent edema
   B. apply elastic bandages and stockings, which should be removed every 4 hours for short periods and reap-plied
   C. assist the patient out of bed within 24 hours, ensuring that elastic stockings are applied
   D. assess for increased bleeding, particularly in the groin area

9. Which of the following would NOT be part of the teaching and discharge planning provided by the nurse to Mrs. Robinson?
   Instruction regarding the

   A. importance of planned rest periods with elevation of the feet
   B. importance of adequate hydration to prevent hyper-coagulability
   C. need to avoid crossing the legs at the knees
   D. use of elastic stockings when on bed rest

10. All of the following statements about *spider veins* are correct EXCEPT:

    A. They are fine, intracutaneous angiectases of no serious consequence, but may be extensive and unsightly
    B. They are mostly symptomatic with patients' common complaints of burning and pain
    C. They can usually be eliminated by intracapillary injections of 1% solution of sodium tetradecyl sulfate through a fine-bore needle
    D. Best results are obtained by treating the whole leg at the initial visit and applying a compression bandage on the leg with ambulation for at least 3 weeks after treatment

Questions 11-18.

DIRECTIONS: Questions 11 through 18 are to be answered on the basis of the following information.

35-year-old Linda Gray comes to the hospital emergency room complaining of dizziness, weakness, and cold sensitivity after having excessive menses.

11. After a careful examination by the physician, Mrs. Gray is diagnosed with iron-deficiency anemia.
    Which of the following statements does NOT provide correct information about this disease?

    A. This is a chronic, microcytic, hypochromic anemia caused by either inadequate absorption or excessive loss of iron.
    B. Acute or chronic bleeding is the principal cause in adults resulting chiefly from trauma, excessive menses, and gastrointestinal bleeding.
    C. It can be caused by chronic diarrhea, malabsorption syndromes, and high cereal product intake with high animal protein ingestion.
    D. In iron-deficiency states, iron stores are depleted first, followed by a reduction in Hgb formation.

12. The incidence of iron-deficiency anemia is related to

    A. geographic location
    B. economic class
    C. age group and sex
    D. all of the above

13. The population affected MOST frequently by iron-deficiency anemia is

    A. women between ages 20-50
    B. men between ages 25-55
    C. children of all ages
    D. women between ages 15-45 and children

14. While assessing Mrs. Gray, the nurse expects to notice all of the following EXCEPT

    A. palpitations, dizziness, and cold sensitivity
    B. brittleness of hair and nails and pallor
    C. dysphagia, pruritis, and atrophic glossitis
    D. dyspnea and weakness

15. Which of the following is NOT a correct laboratory finding for iron-deficiency anemia?

    A. Red blood cells small (microcytic) and pale (hypo-chromic)
    B. Hemosiderin absent from bone marrow
    C. Hgb markedly decreased
    D. Reticulocyte count increased

16. All of the following would be appropriate nursing interventions for Mrs. Gray EXCEPT:

    A. Monitoring for signs and symptoms of bleeding through a hematest of pulmonary contents
    B. Providing for adequate rest and planning activities so as not to overtire
    C. Providing a thorough explanation of all diagnostic tests used to determine sources of possible bleeding, as it helps allay anxiety and ensure cooperation
    D. Monitoring for signs and symptoms of bleeding through a hematest of stool, urine, and gastric contents

17. It would NOT be an appropriate nursing intervention regarding oral iron preparations to

    A. use oral iron preparations as the route of choice, recommended to be given following meals or a snack
    B. dilute liquid preparations well and administer them using a straw to prevent staining teeth
    C. administer with orange juice when possible, as vitamin C (ascorbic acid) enhances iron absorption
    D. warn the patient that iron preparations will make stool color darker and may cause diarrhea

18. Concerning the use of parenteral iron preparations, do NOT

    A. use them in patients intolerant to oral preparations, patients who have no complaints with therapy, or patients who have continuing blood losses
    B. use one needle to withdraw and another to administer iron preparations, as tissue staining and irritation are problems
    C. use the Y track injection technique to prevent leakage into tissues
    D. massage the injection site, but encourage ambulation, as this will enhance absorption; advise against vigorous exercise and constricting garments

Questions 19-30.

DIRECTIONS: Questions 19 through 30 are to be answered on the basis of the following information.

58-year-old John Lithgow is brought to the hospital by his wife after suffering from weakness, sore mouth, diarrhea, and jaundice.

19. After being carefully examined by the physician, John is diagnosed with pernicious anemia, which is correctly explained by all of the following statements EXCEPT:

    A. It is a chronic, progressive, macrocytic anemia caused by a deficiency of intrinsic factor; the result is abnormally large erythrocytes and hypo-chlorhydria
    B. It is characterized by neurologic and gastrointestinal symptoms; death usually results if it goes untreated
    C. A lack of intrinsic factor is caused by gastric mucosal atrophy, possibly due to heredity, prolonged iron deficiency, or an autoimmune disorder
    D. It can result in patients who have had a total gastrec-tomy if vitamin B_2 is not administered

20. It is NOT a true pathophysiological finding about pernicious anemia that

    A. an intrinsic factor is necessary for the absorption of vitamin B_{12} by the large intestine
    B. b_{12} deficiency diminishes DNA synthesis, which results in defective maturation of cells, particularly rapidly dividing cells such as blood cells and gastrointestinal tract cells
    C. B_{12} deficiency can alter structure and function of peripheral nerves
    D. B_{12} deficiency can alter structure and function of the spinal cord and the brain

21. While assessing John, the nurse may expect to notice all of the following EXCEPT   21.____

    A. pallor, dyspnea, palpitations, and fatigue
    B. sore mouth with smooth, beefy, red tongue
    C. tingling, paresthesias of hands and feet and paralysis
    D. depression, hypertension, and psychosis

22. The one of the following that will NOT show up on a laboratory test of pernicious anemia is   22.____

    A. decreased erythrocyte count
    B. blood smear showing oval, macrocytic erythrocytes with a proportionate amount of Hgb
    C. very small numbers of reticulocytes in the blood following parenteral vitamin B_{12} administration
    D. elevated serum LDH

23. Which of the following statements is NOT true about the positive Schilling test? It   23.____

    A. measures absorption of radioactive vitamin B_{12} before parenteral administration of intrinsic factor
    B. measures absorption of radioactive vitamin B_{12} after parenteral administration of extrinsic factor
    C. is a definitive test for pernicious anemia
    D. is used to detect lack of intrinsic factor

24. All of the following will be part of John's drug therapy EXCEPT   24.____

    A. monthly maintenance by vitamin B_{12} injections
    B. iron preparations if Hgb level is inadequate to meet increased number of erythrocytes
    C. folic acid
    D. folic acid, which is safe if given in large amounts in addition to vitamin B_{12}

25. A 1000 mg injection of vitamin B_{12} can be given IM _____ times per week until hematologic abnormalities are corrected; then it is given once monthly.   25.____

    A. 2   B. 3
    C. 4   D. all of the above

26. A nurse should provide all of the following to control John's condition EXCEPT   26.____

    A. mouth care before and after meals using a hard toothbrush for better cleansing and non-irritating rinses
    B. a nutritious diet high in iron, protein, and vitamins such as fish, meat, milk/milk products, and eggs
    C. teaching concerning dietary instructions and the importance of lifelong vitamin B_{12} therapy
    D. bedrest if anemia is severe

27. Folic acid administration to anyone in the B_{12}-deprived state is contraindicated since it may result in fulminant _____ deficit.

    A. renal
    B. hepatic
    C. neurologic
    D. all of the above

28. Pernicious anemia MOST commonly occurs in

    A. men over age 50
    B. women over age 50
    C. blue-eyed persons of Scandinavian descent
    D. all of the above

29. Which of the following statements is FALSE about the Schilling test?

    A. Schilling III can be done after a 2-week trial of oral tetracycline.
    B. Labeled urine collection will contain less than 9% of the administered dose.
    C. Decreased excretion of radiolabeled B_{12} and normal excretion of labeled B_{12} bound to intrinsic factor establishes a defect in intrinsic factor production.
    D. Since the test provides 612 repletion, it should be performed after completion of all studies and planned therapeutic trials.

30. Which of the following is NOT considered a correct laboratory diagnosis finding for pernicious anemia?

    A. The anemia is macrocytic, with an MCV less than 100.
    B. In general, low values of less than 150 pg/mL are reliable indications of vitamin B_{12} deficiency.
    C. In borderline circumstances, i.e., 150-250 pg/mL, clinical judgment and other tests must supplement the radioassay.
    D. Autoantibodies to gastric parietal cells can be identified in 80 to 90% of patients with pernicious anemia and antibodies to intrinsic factor can be found in the sera of most of these patients.

KEY (CORRECT ANSWERS)

1. D
2. D
3. C
4. D
5. D

6. A
7. A
8. B
9. D
10. B

11. C
12. D
13. D
14. C
15. D

16. A
17. D
18. C
19. D
20. A

21. D
22. C
23. B
24. D
25. D

26. A
27. C
28. D
29. B
30. A

TEST 2

DIRECTIONS: Each question or incomplete statement is followed by several suggested answers or completions. Select the one that BEST answers the question or completes the statement. *PRINT THE LETTER OF THE CORRECT ANSWER IN THE SPACE AT THE RIGHT.*

1. In which of the following groups of people is stomach cancer MOST frequently found? 1.___

    A. Spanish
    B. Japanese
    C. White Americans
    D. Black Americans

2. A patient who is severely allergic to penicillin has streptococcal pharyngitis. The drug of choice is 2.___

    A. vancomycin
    B. tetracyline
    C. erythromycin
    D. sulfonamide

3. A 20-year-old male has gonococcal urethritis proven by a culture. The drug of choice to treat him is 3.___

    A. penicillin
    B. erythromycin
    C. ceftriaxon
    D. sulfonamide

4. Hookworm disease can be prevented by 4.___

    A. inspecting meat
    B. washing hands
    C. sterilizing water supply
    D. wearing shoes

5. Pulmonary fibrosis is an adverse side effect of the anti-cancer medication 5.___

    A. adriamycin
    B. vincristin
    C. cyclophosphomide
    D. bleomycin

6. A 25-year-old male is treated with methecillin for staphy-lococcus infection. Ten days later, the patient develops hematuria. The MOST likely diagnosis is 6.___

    A. membrano proliferative glomerulonephritis
    B. acute glomerulonephritis
    C. nephrotic syndrome
    D. allergic nephritis

7. A 20-year-old male's exudative tonsilopharyngitis was treated with ampicillin, after which he developed generalized rash and hepatosplenomaly. What is the MOST likely diagnosis? 7.___

    A. Infectious mononucleosis
    B. Diphtheria
    C. Streptococcal pharyngitis
    D. Hemophilus influenzae pharyngitis

8. A 25-year-old woman has vaginal discharge and her vaginal culture is positive for chlamydia.
   The treatment of choice is

   A. penicillin
   B. metronidazol
   C. erythromycin
   D. amphotericin B

Questions 9-17.

DIRECTIONS: Questions 9 through 17 are to be answered on the basis of the following information.

Sixty-year-old James Bond is brought to the emergency room by his wife after suffering from severe low abdominal and low back pain.

9. After being examined by the physician, Mr. Bond is diagnosed with an abdominal aortic aneurysm, which is BEST defined as a

   A. saccular aneurysm developed above the renal arteries and caused by arteriosclerosis
   B. dissecting aneurysm developed below the iliac bifurcation and caused by atherosclerosis
   C. localized dilation of the aorta developing just above the iliac bifurcation caused by trauma
   D. localized dilation of the abdominal aorta developing just below the renal arteries but above the iliac bifurcation caused by arteriosclerosis, atherosclerosis, hypertension, trauma, syphilis, or other types of infectious processes

10. Abdominal aortic aneurysm occurs MOST often in _____ ages _____.

    A. men; 51-60
    B. women; 51-60
    C. men; 61 and over
    D. women; 61 and over

11. Abdominal aortic aneurysms of arteriosclerosis commonly pass unnoticed until they become large enough to cause symptoms or to be felt as a pulsating mass of about _____ cm.

    A. 2-4   B. 4-6   C. 6-8   D. 8-10

12. While assessing Mr. Bond, the nurse would expect to notice all of the following EXCEPT

    A. severe mid to low abdominal pain and low back pain
    B. mass in the periumbilical area or slightly to the left of the midline with bruits heard over the mass
    C. pulsating abdominal mass
    D. increased femoral pulses

13. _____ is(are) NOT used as a diagnostic test for an abdominal aortic aneurysm.

    A. X-rays
    B. Aortography
    C. Venography
    D. Ultrasound

14. Appropriate pre-operative nursing interventions for abdominal aortic aneurysms include

    A. preparing patient for surgery
    B. assessing rate and rhythm of peripheral pulses
    C. assessing character of the peripheral pulses
    D. all of the above

15. A nurse attending post-operatively to a patient with an abdominal aortic aneurysm does NOT have to

    A. make circulation checks noting rate, rhythm, and character of all pulses distal to the graft at least twice a day
    B. monitor hourly outputs through a Foley catheter
    C. keep the patient flat in bed without sharp flexion of the hip or knee
    D. prevent thrombophlebitis by encouraging the patient to dorsiflex his foot while in bed

16. All of the following would be part of the teaching and discharge planning provided by the nurse to Mr. Bond EXCEPT advice concerning the importance of

    A. changes in color or temperature of extremities
    B. avoidance of prolonged sitting, standing, and smoking
    C. a gradual progressive activity regimen
    D. adherence to a low cholesterol and a high-saturated fat diet

17. The MOST appropriate medical management for Mr. Bond's recovery would be

    A. injection sclerotherapy
    B. clinical monitoring of the indicators of shock
    C. surgical resection of the lesion and replacement with a graft
    D. chlorpromazine 10 to 25 mg orally q 6 to 8 hours

Questions 18-30.

DIRECTIONS: Questions 18 through 30 are to be answered on the basis of the following information.

48-year-old Marge Simpson has been working in a garment factory for the last ten years as a sewing machine operator 8 to 10 hours a day. She comes to the hospital after feeling pain and noticing tenderness and redness in one of her lower extremities. Marge is also a cigarette smoker.

18. After being examined by the physician, Marge is diagnosed with thrombophlebitis, which is BEST defined as the

    A. inflammation of the vessel walls of saphenous and femoral veins with formation of a thrombus
    B. inflammation of the walls of femoral and popliteal veins with formation of an embolus
    C. inflammation of the arterial wall with formation of a thrombus, the most frequently affected arteries being saphenous, femoral, and popliteal
    D. presence of a thrombus in a vein, most commonly in the saphenous, femoral, and popliteal veins

19. Which of the following factors may contribute to thrombophlebitis?

    A. Injury to the epithelium of the vein
    B. Hypercoagulability
    C. Stasis
    D. All of the above

20. The nurse knows that the terms phlegmasia alba dolens and phlegmesia cerulea dolens are applied to extensive thrombosis of the involved extremity depending on

    A. what part of the extremity is involved
    B. size of the involvement
    C. its color
    D. its temperature

21. Effort (strain) thrombosis occurs in the _____ veins, secondary to trauma to the vein in the thoracic outlet during unusual physical effort in which the arm is fully abducted.

    A. esophageal   B. aortic
    C. subclavian   D. pulmonary

22. The nurse would consider all of the following risk factors for Marge EXCEPT

    A. cigarette smoking
    B. intrauterine contraceptive devices
    C. prolonged immobility
    D. complications of surgery

23. The nurse, while assessing Marge, would NOT expect to notice

    A. tenderness, redness, and induration along the course of the vein in the situation of superficial vein involvement
    B. swelling, venous distension of the limb; tenderness and cyanosis in deep veins
    C. elevated WBC and decreased ESR
    D. positive Homan's sign in the situation of deep vein involvement

24. Regarding the anticoagulant therapy used for Marge, it is INCORRECT that

    A. heparin blocks the conversion of prothrombin to thrombin and reduces the formation or extension of thrombus
    B. side effects of heparin include spontaneous bleeding, ecchymosis, cyanosis, thrombocytopenia, and others
    C. warfarin (coumadin) blocks prothrombin synthesis by interfering with vitamin D synthesis
    D. side effects of warfarin include nausea and vomiting, diarrhea, urticaria, pruritis, transient hair loss, burning sensation of feet and others

25. All of the following are true concerning Marge's medical management by surgery EXCEPT:

    A. A good prognosis of vein ligation
    B. A contraindication of vein stripping
    C. Venous thrombectomy; removal of a clot in the ilio-femoral region
    D. Plication of the inferior vena cava; insertion of an umbrella-like prosthesis into the lumen of the vena cava to filter incoming clot

26. _____ would NOT be used as one of the diagnostic tests in the case of Marge.

    A. Venography
    B. Doppler ultrasonography
    C. Plethysmography
    D. The Trendelenburg test

27. A nurse treating Marge would NOT have to

    A. provide bedrest, elevating the involved extremity to increase venous return and decrease edema
    B. apply continuous warm, moist soaks to decrease lymphatic congestion
    C. assess vital signs every 8 hours
    D. monitor for chest pain or shortness of breath

28. When using heparin as an anticoagulant in thrombophlebitis, a nurse should do all of the following EXCEPT

    A. recognize that one of the proper injection techniques is the use of 26- or 27-gauge tuberculin syringe with 1/2 - 5/8 in. needle, injected into the fatty layer of the abdomen below the iliac crest
    B. monitor PTT; dosage should be adjusted to keep PTT between 1.5-2.5 times the normal control level
    C. assess for increased bleeding tendencies and instruct the patient to observe for and report these
    D. have an antidote (protamine sulfate) available

29. All of the following would be appropriate nursing interventions concerning use of warfarin (coumadin) as an anticoagulant in thrombophlebitis EXCEPT

    A. obtaining careful medication history, as there are many drug-drug interactions
    B. instructing patient to use a hard toothbrush and to floss regularly
    C. having an antidote (vitamin K) available
    D. instructing patient to wear Medic-Alert bracelet

30. It would NOT be appropriate teaching and discharge planning for the nurse to tell Marge to

    A. avoid prolonged standing or sitting, constrictive clothing, smoking, and oral contraceptives
    B. avoid physical activities, such as swimming
    C. maintain adequate hydration to prevent hypercoagability
    D. use of elastic stockings when ambulatory

KEY (CORRECT ANSWERS)

1.	B	16.	D
2.	C	17.	C
3.	C	18.	D
4.	D	19.	D
5.	D	20.	C
6.	D	21.	C
7.	A	22.	B
8.	C	23.	C
9.	D	24.	C
10.	C	25.	B
11.	B	26.	D
12.	D	27.	C
13.	C	28.	A
14.	D	29.	B
15.	A	30.	B

EXAMINATION SECTION
TEST 1

DIRECTIONS: Each question or incomplete statement is followed by several suggested answers or completions. Select the one that BEST answers the question or completes the statement. *PRINT THE LETTER OF THE CORRECT ANSWER IN THE SPACE AT THE RIGHT.*

Questions 1-2.

DIRECTIONS: Questions 1 and 2 are to be answered on the basis of the following information.

A 65-year-old man is admitted to the hospital with complaints of difficulty in swallowing food, weight loss of 25 pounds, and loss of appetite.

1. The MOST likely diagnosis is 1._____
    A. achlasia
    B. carcinoma of esophagus
    C. cardiomyopathies
    D. gastritis

2. Regarding the general condition of this patient, gastrostomy has been done as a conservative procedure on this patient. 2._____
   The nurse should follow all of the following principles in the care of the gastrostomy tube EXCEPT:
    A. Be careful about the security of the tube to the dressing so that it won't be kinked
    B. If the patient develops nausea, vomiting or belching, the chances are that he is developing ileus, so a surgeon should be informed
    C. Feeding should be given with the patient in a supine position to prevent regurgitation
    D. Before each feeding, aspiration of gastric contents should be done to see the residual amount

Questions 3-5.

DIRECTIONS: Questions 3 through 5 are to be answered on the basis of the following information.

A 28-year-old truck driver sustains an injury on his left upper abdomen in an accident. Splenic injury is suspected, and he is shifted to the operation theatre for splenectomy.

3. Possible significant findings suggesting hemorrhagic shock in this patient include 3._____
    A. diminished or absent bowel sounds
    B. hypotension (90/50) and rapid and thready pulse
    C. tenderness on left upper abdomen
    D. all of the above

4. The one of the following that is NOT among the serious surgical hazards that can occur in a splenectomy patient is

   A. failure to control bleeding from splenic artery
   B. injury to abdominal aorta
   C. injury to nearby structures, especially pancreas
   D. overlook

5. In an automobile accident like this one, the nurse should be on constant alert for which of the following complications that can occur even 1-2 days after the accident?

   A. Any injury to the chest wall, which can lead to pulmonary contusion manifested as unexplained restlessness, anoxia, and impending respiratory failure
   B. Cerebral injuries that may occur as subdural hematoma, cerebral hemorrhage, and cerebral edema
   C. Any arrhythmia, unexplained hypotension or shock, which suggests cardiac contusion with or without pericardial tamponade
   D. All of the above

Questions 6-8.

DIRECTIONS: Questions 6 through 8 are to be answered on the basis of the following information.

A patient has an appendectomy done for a ruptured appendix.

6. A SIGNIFICANT finding in this patient which may suggest a small bowel obstruction is

   A. fecalent odor to breath
   B. markedly distended abdomen hypertonic on percussion
   C. gas in rectal ampulla
   D. dehydration with dry mucous membrane and loss of tissue turgor

7. This same patient undergoes surgery for lysis of adhesion. During early postoperative management, the nurse.s duties involve all of the following EXCEPT:

   A. Saline should be instilled every 2-3 hours for maintaining potency of long intestinal tube, and it is attached to low intermittent suction
   B. If urine output falls below 26 ml per hour, intravenous fluid infusion should be increased
   C. CVP line should be checked and reading should be taken frequently
   D. If obstruction is relieved and peristalsis resumes, the abdomen should be deflated and fluids started by mouth

8. In a case of a ruptured appendix with generalized peritonitis, nursing intervention in the immediate postoperative period would NOT necessarily include

   A. inspecting wound frequently for swelling, tenderness, and fluctuation, as sepsis is a common occurrence
   B. administering intravenous fluids and intravenous antibiotics
   C. starting feeding 4-8 hours after surgery
   D. putting patient in semi-Fowler's position to encourage drainage of pus into pelvis

Questions 9-12.

DIRECTIONS: Questions 9 through 12 are to be answered on the basis of the following information.

A 65-year-old obese male comes to the clinic with a complaint of intermittent diarrhea and constipation. He also has dull abdominal pain in the left lower region and noted that sometimes his stools are streaked with blood. There is no history of weight loss or anorexia. All of the above symptoms have been present for the last four or five months.

9. What is the MOST likely diagnosis?

    A. Diverticulitis
    B. Carcinoma of colon
    C. Multiple polyposis
    D. Regional enteritis

10. In this type of patient, preparation for surgery begins 4-5 days prior to surgery and includes all of the following EXCEPT

    A. transfusion of packed cells if the patient is anemic
    B. an antibiotic, which should not be absorbed from the gastrointestinal tract and has a broad spectrum activity against colonic bacteria, should be started 24 hours before surgery
    C. high residue diet starting 4-5 days earlier
    D. daily soapsuds enema and laxatives each evening

11. Surgery in such patients is NOT likely to be complicated by

    A. injury to sigmoidal arteries or veins or to the large sacral veins, leading to excessive blood loss
    B. ligation of left ureter, leading to urinary complications
    C. intraperitoneal contamination if the bowel is not adequately prepared
    D. hemorrhagic pancreatitis

12. If a colectomy has been done on this patient, the nurse should be alert for all of the following anticipated complications EXCEPT

    A. in elderly, obese patients, increased incidence of pulmonary embolism
    B. wound infection
    C. acute cholecystitis
    D. pelvic peritonitis

13. _____ does NOT lead to the aggravation of vascular disease.

    A. Hypercholesterolemia
    B. History of hypertension
    C. Diabetes mellitus
    D. Hyperparathyroidism

Questions 14-15.

DIRECTIONS: Questions 14 and 15 are to be answered on the basis of the following information.

A 30-year-old male has a painful, tender, and draining lump over the sacrococcygeal area. The patient is mildly obese and has abundant hairs in his gluteal region.

14. The MOST likely diagnosis is

    A. perianal abscess
    B. fistula in ano
    C. pilonidal cyst
    D. hidradenitis suppurativa

15. Assume this patient undergoes surgery for pilonidal cyst and fistula. In the early postoperative period, the nurse should

    A. watch for acute urinary retention
    B. provide good analgesia as the condition is very painful
    C. give the patient house diet as soon as possible
    D. all of the above

Questions 16-18.

DIRECTIONS: Questions 16 through 18 are to be answered on the basis of the following information.

A 50-year-old, mildly anemic patient comes to the clinic with complaints of rectal bleeding, discomfort, and a feeling of protrusion. He also has a history of mucoid discharge from the rectum. According to the patient, he feels the symptoms especially when he strains at defecation in a squatting position. All of the above symptoms started 4-5 months ago.

16. What may be the cause of this presentation?

    A. Internal hemorrhoids
    B. Carcinoma of colon or rectum
    C. Fistula-in-ano
    D. Ano-rectal abscess

17. If a hemorrhoidectomy is planned for this patient, the nurse should do all of the following in preparation for surgery EXCEPT

    A. keep the patient in a prone position with head down and buttocks separated with tape to expose anal region
    B. wash the perianal region with detergent and paint it with antiseptic to prepare the skin
    C. place Levin tube
    D. give a soapsuds or fleet enema on the morning of surgery

18. In the early postoperative management of this patient, the nurse should be alert for

    A. severe peritonitis
    B. rectal bleeding and acute urinary retention
    C. septicemia
    D. all of the above

Questions 19-22.

DIRECTIONS: Questions 19 through 22 are to be answered on the basis of the following information.

A 55-year-old woman, busy at her daily household chores, suddenly develops severe headache, stiff neck, vomiting, and photophobia. She becomes unconscious and falls to the ground.
Besides these mild to moderate headaches, there is nothing significant in her past history. On neurological examination, no motor or sensory deficit is detectable. Lumbar puncture reveals bloody CSF, and xanthochromic supernatant. CT and angiography are planned.

19. What is the MOST likely diagnosis?   19.____

   A. Subarachnoid hemorrhage secondary to aneurysmal rupture
   B. Subdural hematoma due to fall on the ground
   C. Arteriovenous malformation
   D. Brain tumor

20. Suppose a craniotomy is planned for the clipping of an aneurysm in this patient. In preparing the patient for surgery, the nurse should do all of the following EXCEPT   20.____

   A. provide general information to the patient and her family about the surgical procedure
   B. type and crossmatch six to ten units of blood
   C. routinely do a Levin tube and enema
   D. shave the entire head

21. In the early postoperative management of this patient, which of the following should NOT be done by the nurse?   21.____

   A. Frequent neurological evaluation
   B. Elevating the foot end of the patient
   C. Foley's catheter removed as soon as consciousness is regained
   D. Patient ambulated as soon as her physical and neurological conditions permit

22. The one of the following that is NOT a likely postoperative complication in this patient is   22.____

   A. postoperative hemorrhage
   B. vasospasm of one or more intracranial vessels
   C. arteriovenous malformation
   D. communicating hydrocephalus

Questions 23-25.

DIRECTIONS: Questions 23 through 25 are to be answered on the basis of the following information.

A 38-year-old man develops increasing severity and frequency of chest pain. He has previously had two episodes of myocardial infarction. Now, he has these pain attacks more often, and they hamper his daily chores. He has to take many tablets for the relief of chest pain, which recurs after 2-3 days.

23. This patient has _____ angina.

   A. Prinzmetal's
   B. unstable
   C. stable
   D. hyper

24. If coronary artery bypass surgery is performed on this patient, all of the following surgical complications may occur EXCEPT

   A. arrhythmias
   B. excessive bleeding
   C. cardiac tamponade
   D. cardiomyopathies

25. In the early postoperative management of this patient, the nurse should

   A. maintain adequate ventilation
   B. monitor and control cardiac arrhythmias
   C. maintain fluid and electrolyte balance
   D. all of the above

KEY (CORRECT ANSWERS)

1. B
2. C
3. D
4. B
5. D

6. C
7. B
8. C
9. A
10. C

11. D
12. C
13. D
14. C
15. D

16. A
17. C
18. B
19. A
20. C

21. B
22. C
23. B
24. D
25. D

TEST 2

DIRECTIONS: Each question or incomplete statement is followed by several suggested answers or completions. Select the one that BEST answers the question or completes the statement. *PRINT THE LETTER OF THE CORRECT ANSWER IN THE SPACE AT THE RIGHT.*

Questions 1-4.

DIRECTIONS: Questions 1 through 4 are to be answered on the basis of the following information.

A fifty-year-old female is admitted to the surgical floor with complaints of orthopnea, dyspnea on exertion, peripheral edema and hepatic congestion. She was diagnosed to have rheumatic cardiac disease about 4 years ago. In the course of four years, she was admitted three times for these symptoms. She was previously treated with digoxin and vasodilators, and has had one or two episodes of hemoptysis in the past.

On examination, apical impulse is displaced to the further left side. On auscultation, an apical, high-pitched, holosystolic murmur is heard radiating to the axilla. Imaging techniques show left atrial, left ventricular and right ventricular enlargement along with pulmonary congestion and Kerley B lines.

1. This patient PROBABLY has
    A. mitral insufficiency
    B. aortic insufficiency
    C. tricuspid insufficiency
    D. aortic stenosis

2. Surgical valve replacement is advised on this patient. In the preparation of the patient for surgery, the nurse should
    A. psychologically prepare the patient for surgery
    B. check vital signs frequently and weigh patient daily
    C. enforce a two gram sodium diet and keep a careful record of intake and output
    D. all of the above

3. All of the following are surgical hazards that can occur either on the operation table or immediately in the intensive care unit following the procedure EXCEPT
    A. cardiac arrest
    B. recurrence of the same valvular problem
    C. hemorrhage due to operative trauma or coagulation defect
    D. peripheral embolization due to clots, air or calcium particles broken off during valve replacement

4. In the early postoperative management of this patient, the nurse does NOT have to
    A. monitor vital and neurological signs frequently
    B. watch cardiac rhythm patterns carefully on the monitor for cardiac arrhythmias and measure left atrial and central venous pressure
    C. maintain optimum ventilation by keeping the head of the patient.s bed down and raising the foot end of the bed
    D. maintain optimum renal function by hourly measurement of urine output and specific gravity analysis

5. If renal failure is present after mitral valve replacement, management should consist of all of the following EXCEPT

   A. fluid restriction with careful monitoring of blood electrolytes
   B. control of hypokalemia with use of ion exchange resins
   C. IV administration of insulin, glucose, and sodium bicarbonate
   D. peritoneal and hemodialysis

6. In the neurological evaluation of a patient after surgical valve replacement, in order to determine any neurological deficit the nurse should check

   A. level of consciousness by evaluating the patient's ability to respond to situation, time, place, and person
   B. pupillary reaction to lights and their sizes
   C. change in muscle tone and movements such as drooping eyelids on one side and asymmetrical facial expression
   D. all of the above

7. Implantation of a permanent pacemaker is done on a patient with SKK sinus syndrome. In the early postoperative management of this patient, the nurse should do all of the following EXCEPT

   A. monitor ECG for 24-48 hours after surgery
   B. check for any signs of myocardial perforation and electrode displacement
   C. start IV protamine sulfate
   D. check under dressing for signs of hematoma

Questions 8-10.

DIRECTIONS: Questions 8 through 10 are to be answered on the basis of the following information.

A 64-year-old man comes to the clinic with complaints of breathlessness, cough, hemoptysis, weight loss, fatigue, and anorexia. He is a smoker and has smoked 25-30 cigarettes a day for the last 20 years. Wheezing is also present.

8. Prior to any investigation, the MOST likely diagnosis is

   A. tuberculosis   B. pneumonia
   C. actinomycosis   D. carcinoma of lungs

9. In the early postoperative management of this patient, the nurse should do all of the following EXCEPT

   A. record vital signs every 20 minutes
   B. do chest x-ray studies immediately and the next day after surgery to ensure aeration and re-expansion
   C. stop coughing and deep breathing immediately
   D. elevate head of patient.s bed and change his position from side to side

10. In the chest physiotherapy of the above patient, which should be started 10-12 hours after surgery?

A. Nasotracheal suctioning to promote voluntary coughing
B. Deep endotracheal suctioning to remove thickened secretion if fever and atelectasis persist in spite of aggressive physiotherapy maneuvers
C. Intermittent positive pressure breathing with muco-lytic agents or saline to help loosen tenacious secretions
D. All of the above

11. A _____ does NOT appear on an x-ray as a carcinoma.

    A. hematoma   B. tuberculoma
    C. pneumonia   D. fungus-like mass

12. Surgery is NOT the treatment of choice for a malignant

    A. squamous cell carcinoma   B. bronchial gland carcinoma
    C. small cell carcinoma   D. carcinoid tumor

13. Following most thoracotomies, the surgeon places a chest tube, the advantages of which include

    A. removal or drainage of blood and air from the intra-pleural space
    B. expansion of the lung on the operative side
    C. restoration of sub-atmospheric pressure in the thoracic cavity
    D. all of the above

Questions 14-17.

DIRECTIONS: Questions 14 through 17 are to be answered on the basis of the following information.

A 39-year-old, non-married female noticed a mass in the upper outer quadrant of her left breast, but she didn't pay it much attention. Recently, she noticed an increase in the size of the mass, which is firm and irregular. Besides this, there is nothing else significant in her medical history.

14. The MOST likely diagnosis is

    A. carcinoma of the breast   B. fibroadenoma
    C. fibrocystic disease   D. hematoma

15. The early postoperative management of this patient should include the nurse.s performance of all of the following EXCEPT

    A. keeping the patient in semi-Fowler's position to minimize venous oozing
    B. removing suction catheters from the chest wall 12-24 hours after surgery
    C. starting liquid diet by mouth as soon as the patient is conscious
    D. checking hematocrit to detect any blood loss

16. The BEST technique of diagnostic study for carcinoma of the breast is

    A. open-excisional biopsy
    B. mammography
    C. needle aspiration cystology
    D. ultrasonography

17. A POSSIBLE surgical complication of a radical mastectomy is 17.___
    A. pneumothorax when bleeding vessels are clamped on chest wall
    B. injury to long thoracic nerve or lateral thoracic nerve
    C. injury to brachial plexus and axillary artery, which may result in disability to involved arm
    D. all of the above

Questions 18-19.

DIRECTIONS: Questions 18 and 19 are to be answered on the basis of the following information.

A 28-year-old female enters the hospital with complaints of muscular fatigability, arthralgias, constipation, and bone pain. Previously, she was admitted into the hospital once for ureteral colic. Lab investigation shows hypercalcemia and hypophosphatemia.

18. The BEST diagnosis of this presentation is 18.___
    A. hyperparathyroidism   B. sarcoidosis
    C. multiple myeloma   D. Paget's disease

19. If a parathyroidectomy has been done on this patient, the nurse.s early postoperative management of the patient should include all of the following EXCEPT 19.___
    A. being alert for signs of postoperative tetany by noting paresthesia, tingling, and tremor of extremities
    B. checking for quality of voice after every two hours, as stridor may suggest damage or edema to both laryngeal nerves
    C. checking for signs of hypercalcemia
    D. ensuring that suction apparatus and a tracheostomy kit are available at all times

20. Blood is NOT supplied to the thyroid gland by the 20.___
    A. thyroidea ima
    B. superior thyroid artery
    C. middle thyroid artery
    D. inferior thyroid artery

Questions 21-24.

DIRECTIONS: Questions 21 through 24 are to be answered on the basis of the following information.

A 44-year-old male comes to the clinic with a complaint of weight loss in spite of good appetite. On examination, you find warm hands, increased pulse rate, and a large mass in the neck.

21. The FIRST lab investigation the doctor orders will probably be a

    A. radioactive iodine test
    B. serum T_3 and T_4
    C. TSI measurement
    D. serum cholesterol determination

22. Further investigation diagnoses it to be a case of toxic nodular goiter. Thyroidectomy is planned. In order to prepare this patient for surgery,

    A. he should be prepared psychologically by providing good emotional support
    B. antithyroid drug should be started and surgery planned as soon as he becomes euthyroid
    C. 10-15 days before surgery, Lugol's iodine solution should be given to decrease vascularity of gland
    D. all of the above

23. Which of the following is NOT among the surgical hazards of thyroidectomy?

    A. Damage to facial nerve
    B. Damage to one or both recurrent laryngeal nerves
    C. Severe uncontrolled hemorrhage
    D. Damage to parathyroid gland

24. If the patient develops laryngeal edema and stridor, management would include all of the following EXCEPT

    A. rapidly inserting an endotracheal tube
    B. starting IV antibiotics
    C. acting quickly to prevent anoxia and resulting cardiac arrest
    D. administering humidified oxygen by mask

25. Parathyroid glands embryologically develop from the pharyngeal pouch(es)

    A. I   B. II   C. III and IV   D. V

KEY (CORRECT ANSWERS)

1. A
2. D
3. B
4. C
5. B

6. D
7. C
8. D
9. C
10. D

11. C
12. C
13. D
14. A
15. B

16. A
17. D
18. A
19. C
20. C

21. B
22. D
23. A
24. B
25. C

EXAMINATION SECTION
TEST 1

DIRECTIONS: Each question or incomplete statement is followed by several suggested answers or completions. Select the one that BEST answers the question or completes the statement. *PRINT THE LETTER OF THE CORRECT ANSWER IN THE SPACE AT THE RIGHT.*

Questions 1-2.

DIRECTIONS: Questions 1 and 2 are to be answered on the basis of the following information.

Mrs. Smith, 34 years old, is admitted to the hospital after an automobile accident. She has a fractured hip and is taken to surgery for repair. On return from surgery, Mrs. Smith is very much concerned about her obesity.

1. Mrs. Smith asks the nurse how she should lose weight. The nurse's BEST reply would be to tell her that 1.____

    A. fats should be limited in her diet
    B. she needs to exercise vigorously no matter what she eats
    C. her eating pattern should be altered with all 4 basic groups and include light exercise
    D. only carbohydrates have to be completely stopped

2. The physician ordered non-weight bearing with crutches for Mrs. Smith. What should the nurse advise her regarding walking with crutches? 2.____

    A. To strengthen the muscles, exercise them, using triceps, finger flexors, and elbow extensors
    B. Sitting up in a chair strengthens back muscles
    C. The head and neck muscles should be exercised
    D. None of the above

Questions 3-7.

DIRECTIONS: Questions 3 through 7 are to be answered on the basis of the following information.

John, a factory worker, is admitted to the hospital for mild chest pain. A myocardial infarct is diagnosed. The physician orders morphine sulphate, diazepam, and lidocaine.

3. John asks the nurse why he is being given morphine sulphate. The nurse should tell him that morphine sulphate 3.____

    A. relieves pain associated with myocardial infarction
    B. decreases apprehension
    C. prevents cardiogenic shock
    D. all of the above

4. The patient is also prescribed oxygen by nasal cannula. The nurse takes safety precautions in the room because oxygen

   A. converts to an alternate form of matter
   B. supports combustion
   C. has unstable properties
   D. is flammable

5. In a case of myocardial infarction, the finding on the electrocardiogram should be

   A. disappearance of Q waves
   B. absent P wave
   C. elevated ST segments
   D. flattened T waves

6. Several days after admission, John develops pyrexia.
   The nurse should monitor him for

   A. dyspnea   B. increased pulse rate
   C. chest pain   D. elevated blood pressure

7. John asks the nurse about the chances of his having another heart attack if he watches his diet and stress level.
   The nurse should

   A. tell him he is at no risk
   B. suggest that he talk to a psychiatric nurse for his fear about this
   C. avoid giving him direct information
   D. none of the above

Questions 8-10.

DIRECTIONS: Questions 8 through 10 are to be answered on the basis of the following information.

Mrs. Allbright is 65 years old and is suspected to have pernicious anemia.

8. The first test ordered is a Schillings test.
   The nurse should know that the purpose of this test is to check the person's ability to _____ vitamin B _____.

   A. absorb; 12   B. digest; 12
   C. absorb; 6   D. store; 1

9. The nurse should explain the therapeutic regimen for pernicious anemia to Mrs. Allbright as consisting of

   A. oral tablets of B_{12} daily
   B. IM injections daily
   C. IM injections once a month
   D. oral tablets every week

10. Mrs. Allbright wants to know how long she will need therapy. 10.____
    The nurse should reply that she will need therapy

    A. when she feels fatigued
    B. for the rest of her life
    C. until her symptoms subside
    D. during exacerbations of anemia

Questions 11-16.

DIRECTIONS: Questions 11 through 16 are to be answered on the basis of the following information.

Mr. Roberts is 45 years old. He is brought to the emergency room after a terrible motor vehicle accident in which he received multiple crushing wounds of the chest, abdomen, and legs. His right leg might have to be amputated.

11. Upon arrival, the nursing staff's FIRST priority should be to assess 11.____

    A. blood pressure
    B. pain
    C. quality of respiration and presence of pulse
    D. level of consciousness

12. Mr. Roberts' condition requires endotracheal intubation and positive pressure ventilation. 12.____
    The IMMEDIATE nursing intervention should be to

    A. facilitate verbal communication
    B. assess his response to the equipment
    C. maintain sterility of ventilation system
    D. prepare for emergency surgery

13. A chest tube with water seal drainage is inserted. The chest tube seems obstructed. 13.____
    The MOST appropriate nursing action at this time would be to

    A. clamp tube immediately
    B. remove chest tube
    C. milk the tube toward collection container
    D. take a chest x-ray

14. What is the function of the chest tube placed in Mr. Roberts? 14.____
    To

    A. normalize intrathoracic pressure
    B. drain fluid from pleural space
    C. drain air from pleural space
    D. all of the above

15. A response that would indicate that Mr. Roberts' condition was improving is 15.____

    A. increased breath sounds
    B. constant bubbling in drainage chamber
    C. increased respiratory rate
    D. crepitus on palpation of chest

16. In Mr. Roberts' case, adequate tissue perfusion to vital organs would be indicated by

    A. central venous pressure of 2 cm H_2O
    B. urinary output of 30 ml in an hour
    C. pulse rate of 120-110 in 15 minutes
    D. blood pressure of 50/30 and 70/40 in 30 minutes

17. A 47-year-old man is brought into the emergency room following an accident. He has severe abdominal pain in the left upper quadrant. Splenic rupture is diagnosed, and an emergency splenectomy is to be performed.
    The nurse should tell the patient

    A. about the presence of abdominal drains several days after surgery
    B. that splenectomy has a low mortality rate (5%), except with multiple injuries
    C. not to worry about bleeding as it occurs more frequently with repairs than removal
    D. all of the above

Questions 18-19.

DIRECTIONS: Questions 18 and 19 are to be answered on the basis of the following information.

A 34-year-old woman was involved in an accident as a result of which her left leg had to be amputated below the knee. After the operation, the patient refused to talk, eat, or perform any activities.

18. The BEST nursing approach in this case would be to

    A. appear cheerful, regardless of the patient's condition
    B. force her to do exercises
    C. accept and acknowledge that withdrawal is an initially normal and necessary part of grieving
    D. emphasize that nothing has changed in her life and she can and should resume normal life

19. The factors responsible for this change in this patient include the _____ of the change.

    A. client's perception
    B. suddenness
    C. extent
    D. all of the above

20. In dealing with a terminally ill patient who is in the denial stage of grief, the BEST nursing approach is to

    A. encourage the patient's denial
    B. reassure the patient that everything will be okay
    C. allow denial but be available to discuss death
    D. leave the patient alone

Questions 21-25.

DIRECTIONS: Questions 21 through 25 are to be answered on the basis of the following information

A 62-year-old patient is admitted to the coronary care unit with a diagnosis of left-sided congestive heart failure.

21. The findings in this case would MOST likely include   21.____

    A. dyspnea on exertion
    B. chest pain of the crushing type
    C. peripheral edema
    D. jugular vein distention

22. This patient was ordered a cardiac glycoside, a vasodilator, and furosemide (lasix).   22.____
    The site of effect of furosemide is the

    A. collecting tube   B. ascending loop of Henle
    C. distil tube   D. glomerulus

23. The distil tube is the site of action of   23.____

    A. thiazides   B. triamtere
    C. xanthines   D. spironolactone

24. Cardiac glycosides, such as digitalis, _____ the conduction speed in the myocardium   24.____
    and _____ the heart rate.

    A. increase; slow down   B. increase; speed up
    C. decrease; slow down   D. decrease; speed up

25. In cases of congestive heart failure, the nurse should suggest a dietary restriction of   25.____

    A. potassium   B. sodium   C. magnesium   D. iron

KEY (CORRECT ANSWERS)

1. C   11. C
2. A   12. B
3. D   13. C
4. B   14. D
5. C   15. A

6. B   16. B
7. C   17. D
8. A   18. C
9. C   19. D
10. B   20. C

            21. A
            22. B
            23. A
            24. C
            25. B

TEST 2

DIRECTIONS: Each question or incomplete statement is followed by several suggested answers or completions. Select the one that BEST answers the question or completes the statement. *PRINT THE LETTER OF THE CORRECT ANSWER IN THE SPACE AT THE RIGHT.*

1. While taking a history of a patient with G.I. bleeding, the nurse should put the MOST emphasis on

    A. family history
    B. socioeconomic history
    C. history of any recent medications such as aspirin or prednisone
    D. travel of an endemic area

    1.___

2. What kind of dietary management is APPROPRIATE for a patient with gastric ulceration to prevent the mucosal lining from the adverse effects of acids?

    A. Three meals a day
    B. Regular meals and snacks to relieve gastric discomfort
    C. One meal a day
    D. Eat whenever hungry

    2.___

3. Precautions that should be taken by a nurse in order to prevent infections from an indwelling catheter include

    A. changing the bag periodically and not emptying it
    B. maintaining the ordered hydration which flushes the bladder and prevents infection
    C. collecting specimens in order to check for infection
    D. all of the above

    3.___

Questions 4-7.

DIRECTIONS: Questions 4 through 7 are to be answered on the basis of the following information.

Mr. Connery, a 65-year-old patient, is scheduled for surgery of transurethral resection of the prostate.

4. The nurse should let Mr. Connery know that after surgery

    A. his urinary control may be completely lost
    B. urinary drainage will be by a catheter for 24-48 hours
    C. everything will be completely normal
    D. his ability to perform sexually will be completely impaired

    4.___

5. In Mr. Connery's case, the MOST common complication following surgery is

    A. hemorrhage
    B. sepsis
    C. urinary retention with overflow
    D. none of the above

    5.___

6. 24 hours after surgery, Mr. Connery, who is still on a catheter, complains of lower abdominal discomfort. The nurse notices that catheter drainage has stopped.
   The nurse's NEXT step should be to

   A. remove the catheter
   B. notify the physician
   C. irrigate with saline
   D. milk the catheter tubing

7. Which of the following discharge instructions given by the nurse is MOST important for Mr. Connery?

   A. Void at least every 3 hours
   B. Avoid exercise for 6 months after surgery
   C. Call the physician if urinary stream decreases
   D. Get 18 hours of sleep every 24 hours

Questions 8-10.

DIRECTIONS: Questions 8 through 10 are to be answered on the basis of the following information.

Mrs. Ford is admitted to the hospital for a subtotal thyroidectomy. She has a history of Grave's disease.

8. It is important that the nurse know that in a subtotal thyroidectomy

   A. the entire thyroid gland is removed
   B. a small part is left intact
   C. part of the parathyroid is also removed
   D. only parathyroids are removed

9. Classical signs of hyperthyroidism include

   A. weight loss
   B. exopthalmos
   C. restlessness
   D. all of the above

10. Signs of postsurgical hypothyroidism of which Mrs. Ford should be aware include

    A. intolerance to heat
    B. weight loss
    C. dry skin and fatigue
    D. insomnia

Questions 11-13.

DIRECTIONS: Questions 11 through 13 are to be answered on the basis of the following information.

Lisa, a 32-year-old woman, is admitted for treatment of partial and full thickness burns on the lower half of her body. She is in pain.

11. The nurse applies sulphamylon cream to Lisa's burns. This will

    A. relieve the pain
    B. inhibit bacterial growth

C. provide debridement
D. prevent scar tissue formation

12. Pig skin temporary grafts are used for Lisa's burns. The grafts will

    A. relieve the pain
    B. promote rapid epethelialization
    C. provide a framework for granulation
    D. all of the above

13. Lisa suffers from periodic episodes of dyspnea.
    The BEST position for her is the _____ position.

    A. orthopheic   B. sims
    C. semi-fowler's   D. supine

Questions 14-17.

DIRECTIONS: Questions 14 through 17 are to be answered on the basis of the following information.

Mrs. Hunt is 61 years old. She has a history of hypertension over the past 15 years. She complains of dyspnea and pedal edema.

14. The dyspnea is PROBABLY due to

    A. asthma
    B. left ventricular failure
    C. wheezing and coughing
    D. none of the above

15. Mrs. Hunt has been prescribed hydrochlorothiazide.
    A COMMON side effect of this drug is

    A. insomnia
    B. increased thirst
    C. generalized weakness due to hypokalemia
    D. increased muscle strength as a result of hypercalcemia

16. Mrs. Hunt has also been prescribed a potassium supplement because of the diuretic she is taking.
    Potassium supplements

    A. are completely harmless
    B. should not be taken on an empty stomach as they cause GI ulceration and bleeding
    C. possess no side effects at all
    D. all of the above

17. The nurse should tell Mrs. Hunt to

    A. rest during the day to decrease the demand on her heart
    B. sleep with her head slightly elevated to facilitate respiration

C. take her pulse just once daily
D. all of the above

Questions 18-20.

DIRECTIONS: Questions 18 through 20 are to be answered on the basis of the following information.

Mr. Edwards had a partial nephrectomy done and is admitted with a nephrostomy tube in place.

18. The MOST common life-threatening complication in the early post-operative period is 18.____

    A. sepsis
    B. hemorrhage
    C. renal failure
    D. none of the above

19. The nurse's post-operative plan for Mr. Edwards should include 19.____

    A. turning him from back to operated site to facilitate drainage
    B. keeping him on clear fluid for 24-48 hours
    C. draining dressing frequently
    D. all of the above

20. Upon discharge, Mr. Edwards, who is being discharged with nephrostomy tube in place, should be instructed to 20.____

    A. change dressings frequently
    B. limit fluid intake
    C. maintain bedrest at home
    D. all of the above

21. Mrs. Beatty comes to the clinic with complaints of increased appetite, thirst, and weight loss despite more eating. She is diagnosed with diabetes mellitus, and the doctor prescribed her an oral hypoglycemic. 21.____
    The MOST common side effect of oral hypoglycemic agents is

    A. diabetic coma
    B. weight loss
    C. hypoglycemia
    D. all of the above

Questions 22-25.

DIRECTIONS: Questions 22 through 25 are to be answered on the basis of the following information.

Mr. Mailer, a 34-year-old executive, is diagnosed with a peptic ulcer.

22. The pain of a peptic ulcer is COMMONLY described as 22.____

    A. dull pain in the shoulder
    B. gnawing and boring in the epigastrium and back
    C. sharp pain in the abdomen
    D. heartburn upon lying down

23. The physician prescribes ranitidine for Mr. Mailer. Ranitidine

   A. can be given PO, IV, or IM
   B. is usually given with meals
   C. reduces gastric acid in the stomach
   D. all of the above

24. Mr. Mailer's condition worsens while in the hospital. He vomited and complained of severe epigastric pain. His pulse is 134, respiration is 32/minute, and there is an absence of bowel sounds. The nurse calls for the physician.
   The NEXT step should be to

   A. keep the client NPO in preparation for possible surgery
   B. start oxygen
   C. place the client in the Trendelenberg position
   D. all of the above

25. A subtotal gastrectomy (Billroth 1) is performed on Mr. Mailer. He starts eating more food, but he experiences cramping discomfort and rapid pulse with waves of weakness followed by nausea and vomiting.
   The nurse recognizes that Mr. Mailer is going through a *dumping syndrome* caused by the _____ into the small intestine.

   A. slow passage of food dumping
   B. rapid passage of food (hyperosmolar)
   C. rapid passage of dilute food
   D. none of the above

KEY (CORRECT ANSWERS)

1. C	11. B
2. B	12. D
3. D	13. A
4. B	14. B
5. A	15. C
6. D	16. B
7. C	17. D
8. B	18. B
9. D	19. D
10. C	20. A

21. C
22. B
23. D
24. A
25. B

EXAMINATION SECTION
TEST 1

DIRECTIONS: Each question or incomplete statement is followed by several suggested answers or completions. Select the one that BEST answers the question or completes the statement. *PRINT THE LETTER OF THE CORRECT ANSWER IN THE SPACE AT THE RIGHT.*

1. Immediately after delivery, the neonate must assume the life-support functions performed by the placenta in utero. Birth begins a critical 24-hour phase which encompasses the neonate's adaptation from intrauterine to extrauterine life.
   This phase is called the _____ period.

   A. conversion
   B. translocation
   C. uterine adaptation
   D. transitional

2. To survive outside the womb, the neonate must successfully go through the period of adaptation from intrauterine to extrauterine life. Mortality is higher during this period than at any other time.
   Two-thirds of all neonatal deaths occur in the first _____ week(s) after birth.

   A. one   B. two   C. three   D. four

3. Crucial physiologic adjustments take place in all body systems after birth.
   The _____ system(s) undergo(es) IMMEDIATE drastic changes as soon as the umbilical cord is clamped and respiration begins.

   A. pulmonary
   B. hematologic
   C. cardiovascular
   D. pulmonary and cardiovascular

4. To ensure the neonate's survival, fetal circulation must convert to neonatal circulation during the _____ period.

   A. conversion
   B. translocation
   C. uterine adaptation
   D. transitional

5. Fetal circulation involves all of the following unique anatomic features that shunt most blood away from the liver and lungs EXCEPT the

   A. placenta
   B. ductus arteriosus and ductus venosus
   C. pulmonary trunk
   D. foramen ovale

6. Which of the following statements does NOT give correct information about the functions of anatomic features involved in the fetal circulation?
   The

   A. placenta serves as an exchange organ through which the fetus absorbs oxygen, nutrients, and other substances and excretes wastes such as carbon dioxide
   B. ductus venosus links the inferior vena cava with the umbilical vein, permitting most placental blood to bypass the liver

C. foramen ovale directs most blood away from the pulmonary ovale
D. ductus arteriosus directs most blood towards the pulmonary circuit

7. Onset of respiratory effort and the effects of increased partial pressure of arterial oxygen (PaO$_2$) constrict the ductus arteriosus, which functionally closes 15 to 24 hours after birth.
   This shunt undergoes anatomic closure by the age of _____ weeks.

   A. 1 to 2   B. 2 to 3   C. 3 to 4   D. 4 to 5

8. Clamping of the umbilical cord halts blood flow through the ductus venosus, closing this structure.
   The ductus venosus closes anatomically by the _____ week.

   A. first or second   B. second or third
   C. third or fourth   D. fourth or fifth

9. Because anatomic closure lags behind functional closure, fetal shunts may open intermittently before closing completely. Intermittent shunt opening most commonly stems from conditions causing increased vena caval and right atrial pressure, such as crying. Also, because shunts allow unoxygenated blood to pass from the right to the left side of the heart, bypassing the pulmonary circuit, they may cause

   A. atrial septal defects
   B. transient cyanosis
   C. ventricular septal defects
   D. pulmonic stenosis

10. Depending on the amount of blood transferred from the placenta after delivery, the blood volume of the full-tern neonate ranges from _____ ml/kg of body weight.

    A. 60 to 70   B. 70 to 80   C. 80 to 90   D. 90 to 100

11. Delayed umbilical cord clamping may cause all of the following EXCEPT

    A. increase in blood volume by up to 100 ml
    B. increased heart rate and respiratory rate
    C. decreased systolic blood pressure
    D. changes caused by increased blood volume may persist for about 48 hours, possibly leading to crackles and cyanosis

12. Which of the following statements gives CORRECT information about the fetal respiratory system?

    A. Between weeks 25 and 30 of gestation, Type II pneumo-cytes begin limited secretion of surfactant
    B. A phospholipid surfactant decreases the surface tension of pulmonary fluids and prevents alveolar collapse at the end of expiration
    C. Reduction of surface tension facilitates gas exchange, decreases inflation pressures needed to open the airways, improves lung compliance, and decreases labor of breathing
    D. All of the above

13. The fetal lungs contain fluid secreted by the lungs, amniotic cavity, and trachea. The fluid volume, which correlates with the neonate's functional residual capacity (FRC), typically reaches how many ml/kg of body weight?

    A. 50 to 45 B. 35 to 40 C. 30 to 25 D. 15 to 20

14. After respiration begins in a neonate, most of the lung fluid is removed through the

    A. pulmonary circulation and lymphatic system
    B. mouth
    C. nose
    D. all of the above

15. After vaginal delivery of a healthy and full-term neonate, the time needed to clear the lungs varies from _____ hours.

    A. 6 to 20 B. 8 to 16 C. 6 to 24 D. 8 to 32

16. Inadequate lung fluid removal may cause _____ in neonates.

    A. epiglottitis B. pneumonia
    C. cystic fibrosis D. transient tachypnea

17. Stimulated by the medullary respiratory center, the neonate normally breathes within _____ seconds after delivery.

    A. 15 B. 20 C. 25 D. 30

18. _____ provides the STRONGEST stimulus for the first breath in a neonate.

    A. Hypoxemia B. Hypercapnia
    C. Acidosis D. Asphyxia

19. The respiratory rate varies over the first day, stabilizing by about 24 hours after birth. Maintained by the effects of biochemical and environmental stimulation, all of the following are important factors required for the neonate's respiratory function EXCEPT

    A. a patent airway and a functioning respiratory center
    B. intact nerves from the brain to the chest muscles
    C. intact vessels from the heart to the thoracic muscles
    D. adequate calories to supply energy for labor of breathing

20. Which of the following is NOT correct about the neonatal hematopoietic system?

    A. Erythropoiesis is stimulated by the renal hormone erythropoietin. In the fetus, low oxygen saturation causes erythropoietin release to rise; to ensure adequate tissue oxygenation, red blood cell production increases. At birth, the increased oxygen saturation that follows the onset of respiration inhibits erythropoietin release, reducing red blood cell production.
    B. Fetal red blood cells have a life span of about 60 days, compared to 120 days for normal red blood cells.
    C. As fetal red blood cells deteriorate, the neonate's red blood cell count decreases, sometimes resulting in physiologic anemia before stabilization.
    D. By age 2 to 3 months, the red blood cell count rises to within acceptable neonatal limits.

21. All of the following are correct about neonatal white blood cells EXCEPT:

    A. White blood cells, which serve as the neonate's major defense against infection, exist in five types, i.e., neutrophils, eosinophils, basophils, lymphocytes, and monocytes.
    B. Neutrophils account for 40% to 80% of total white blood cells at birth.
    C. Lymphocytes account for roughly 10% of total white blood cells at birth; however, by age 1 month, lymphocytes outnumber neutrophils.
    D. Neutrophils and monocytes are phagocytes, forming part of the mononuclear phagocytic system, which defends the body against infection and disposes of cell breakdown products.

22. The neonate usually has an adequate platelet count and function. Thrombocytes are crucial to

    A. bilirubin metabolism
    B. carbohydrate metabolism
    C. iron storage
    D. blood coagulation

23. The neonate's hepatic system is responsible for

    A. bilirubin clearance and iron storage
    B. blood coagulation
    C. carbohydrate metabolism
    D. all of the above

24. All of the following are correct about bilirubin clearance mechanism in the neonate's body EXCEPT:

    A. Bilirubin is a by-product of heme after red blood cell breakdown. As red blood cells age, they become fragile and eventually are cleared from the circulation by the mononuclear phagocytic system.
    B. After leaving the mononuclear phagocytic system, bilirubin binds to plasma albumin, resulting in a water-insoluble state, and is called the indirect or unconjugated bilirubin.
    C. Indirect bilirubin must be conjugated for excretion. Conjugation occurs in the liver as bilirubin combines with glucuronic acid with the assistance of the enzyme glucuronyl transferase, resulting in a water-soluble state.
    D. The whole portion of the bilirubin compounds resulting from breakdown, called urobilinogen and sterco-bilinogen, is typically excreted in the urine.

25. Factors that may increase the risk of unconjugated hyper-bilirubinemia do NOT include

    A. cold stress and alkalosis
    B. asphyxia
    C. hypoglycemia
    D. maternal salicylate ingestion

KEY (CORRECT ANSWERS)

1. A
2. D
3. D
4. D
5. C

6. D
7. C
8. A
9. B
10. C

11. C
12. D
13. C
14. A
15. C

16. D
17. B
18. D
19. C
20. B

21. C
22. D
23. D
24. D
25. A

TEST 2

DIRECTIONS: Each question or incomplete statement is followed by several suggested answers or completions. Select the one that BEST answers the question or completes the statement. *PRINT THE LETTER OF THE CORRECT ANSWER IN THE SPACE AT THE RIGHT.*

1. Of the following, _____ jaundice is NOT considered a type of jaundice that occurs in the neonate. 1.___

    A. physiologic
    B. pathologic
    C. formula-feeding-associated
    D. breastfeeding-associated

2. All of the following are true facts about physiologic jaundice in neonates EXCEPT: 2.___

    A. It arises 48 to 72 hours after birth.
    B. The serum bilirubin level peaks at 4 to 12 mg/dl by the third to fifth day after birth. On average, the bilirubin level increases by less than 5 mg/dl/day.
    C. It normally disappears by the end of the twelfth day.
    D. Five conditions that may cause physiologic jaundice include decreased hepatic circulation, increased bilirubin load, reduced hepatic bilirubin uptake from the plasma, decreased bilirubin conjugation, and decreased bilirubin excretion.

3. Which of the following statements gives CORRECT information about pathologic jaundice in neonates? 3.___

    A. It occurs within the first 24 hours after birth
    B. The serum bilirubin level rises above 13 mg/dl
    C. It may stem from conditions such as blood group or blood type incompatibilities; hepatic, biliary or metabolic abnormalities; or infection
    D. All of the above

4. All of the following are true findings about breast milk jaundice (BMJ) EXCEPT: 4.___

    A. BMJ appears as physiologic jaundice subsides. Among various suggested causes, current theory focuses on increased breast milk levels of the enzyme beta-glucuronidase which is believed to cause increased intestinal bilirubin absorption in the neonate, thus blocking bilirubin's excretion.
    B. The serum bilirubin level peaks at 15 to 25 mg/dl between days 10 and 15.
    C. BMJ disappears within 3 to 4 weeks.
    D. A serum bilirubin level that decreases 24 to 48 hours after discontinuation of breastfeeding confirms the diagnosis.

5. Which of the following is NOT a fact related to breast-feeding-associated jaundice (BFAJ)? 5.___

    A. The underlying cause of BFAJ is poor caloric intake that leads to decreased hepatic transport and removal of bilirubin from the body. Typically, the neonate who develops BFAJ has not been able to stimulate an early and adequate supply of breast milk.
    B. BFAJ appears 72 to 96 hours after birth.

C. The serum bilirubin level peaks at 15 to 19 mg/dl by 72 hours. The average serum bilirubin level increases by less than 5 mg/dl/day. If the bilirubin level approaches 18 to 20 mg/dl, phototherapy may be necessary.
D. Treatment of BFAJ involves measures that ensure an adequate breast milk supply. Wilkerson recommends breastfeeding the neonate every 2 hours to stimulate the mother's milk production and the neonate's intestinal motility.

6. To assess the risk for bilirubin encephalopathy (kernic-terus), a life-threatening condition characterized by bilirubin deposition in the basal ganglia of the brain, the neonate's condition and gestational and chronological ages must be considered in conjunction with the bilirubin level.
   _____ serum bilirubin levels of approximately _____mg/dl or higher may lead to bilirubin encephalopathy, and may be treated with _____.

   A. Unconjugated; 20; phototherapy or exchange transfusions
   B. Conjugated; 20; phototherapy or exchange transfusions
   C. Indirect; 10; phototherapy
   D. Direct; 10; exchange transfusions

   6.____

7. For the first few days after birth, the gastrointestinal tract lacks the bacterial action to synthesize adequate vitamin K.
   Vitamin K catalyzes synthesis of prothrombin by the liver, thereby activating all of the following coagulation factors EXCEPT Factor

   A. III   B. VII   C. IX   D. X

   7.____

8. Glucose, which is the major energy source during the first 4 to 6 hours after birth, is stored in the liver as

   A. dextrose   B. galactose
   C. glutemic acid   D. glycogen

   8.____

9. If the neonate does not receive exogenous glucose, glycogenolysis occurs.
   Until the neonate takes in sufficient glucose, glycogenolysis causes release of sufficient glucose into the bloodstream to maintain a serum glucose level of approximately _____ mg/dl.

   A. 30   B. 60   C. 50   D. 40

   9.____

10. Provided the mother ingested adequate iron during her pregnancy, by term, the liver contains enough iron to produce red blood cells until about age _____ months

    A. 3   B. 4   C. 5   D. 6

    10.____

11. In the last trimester of pregnancy, the fetal kidneys undergo tremendous growth and maturation. At 34 weeks of gestation, the glomerular filtration rate (GFR) and, consequently, renal function improve markedly.
    The GFR reaches 30% of adult values within the first 2 days of extrauterine life, but it does not attain full adult values until about the age of

    A. 6 months   B. 1 year   C. 2 years   D. 3 years

    11.____

12. All of the following are correct about the neonate's body fluid balance EXCEPT:

    A. At birth, water makes up approximately 70% of the body composition, compared to approximately 58% by adulthood.
    B. Extracellular fluid accounts for about 40% of the neonate's total body water, compared to about 20% by adulthood.
    C. Loss of fluid through urine, feces, insensible losses, intake restrictions related to small gastric capacity, and increased metabolic rate contribute to a reduction of 5% to 15% of the birth weight over the first five days of extrauterine life.
    D. The neonate should regain the birth weight within five days.

13. The birth weight of an infant TYPICALLY doubles by age _____ months and triples by _____.

    A. 5 to 6; the first birthday
    B. 6 to 7; age 18 months
    C. 7 to 8; the second birthday
    D. none of the above

14. All of the following are correct about a neonate's gastric capacity EXCEPT:

    A. Because of a relatively immature GI system, even a healthy neonate can not ingest, absorb, and digest nutrients well.
    B. Gastric capacity is between 40 and 60 ml on the first day after birth, which increases with subsequent feedings.
    C. Gastric emptying time, which is typically 2 to 4 hours, varies with the volume of the feeding and the neonate's age. Peristalsis is rapid.
    D. Many neonates regurgitate a small amount of ingested matter, i.e., 1 to 2 ml after feedings, because of an immature cardiac sphincter, which is a muscular ring constricting the esophagus.

15. Which of the following statements is NOT true with regard to the neonate's GI enzymes?

    A. Compared to the adult's intestine, the neonate's is longer relative to body size and has more secretory glands and a larger absorptive surface.
    B. The stomach lining consists of chief cells, which secrete pepsinogen and promote protein digestion, and parietal cells, which secrete hydrochloric acid to maintain gastric acidity.
    C. Salivary glands secrete only minimal amounts of saliva until age 5 to 6 months, when drooling becomes apparent.
    D. Milk digestion begins in the stomach and continues in the small intestine. Secretions from the pancreas, liver, and duodenum aid digestion.

16. Synthesis of vitamin K through bacterial action is an important GI function. Although initially sterile, the neonate's GI tract establishes normal colonic bacteria, allowing adequate vitamin K synthesis within _____ after birth.

    A. 48 hours   B. 1 week   C. 2 weeks   D. 3 weeks

17. In most cases, feeding should begin as soon as the neonate is physiologically stable and exhibits adequate coordination of the sucking and swallowing reflexes.
An extended delay before feedings may deplete the neonate's limited glycogen reserves, which are already taxed by the increased energy demands of the transitional period, resulting in

   A. hypogalactocemia
   B. hypogammaglobulinemia
   C. hypogeusia
   D. hypoglycemia

17._____

18. Which of the following is an INCORRECT statement about the neonate's urine?

   A. The neonate usually voids within 24 hours of birth. The first urine may be dark red and cloudy from urate and mucus with slight reddish stain of no clinical significance.
   B. The neonate's urine usually is odorless, with specific gravity ranging from 1.005 to 1.015.
   C. Gradually, with increased urine output due to an increase in the neonate's fluid intake, urine becomes clear or light straw in color. The breastfed neonate may require 4 to 8 diaper changes daily.
   D. The bottle-fed neonate typically requires about 6 diaper changes daily.

18._____

19. All of the following are correct statements about neonatal stools that a nurse should know for better neonatal care EXCEPT:

   A. Initially, the neonate's intestines contain meconium, a thick, dark green, odorless fecal substance consisting of amniotic fluid, bile, epithelial cells, and hair. Typically, the neonate passes the first meconium stool within 24 hours of birth.
   B. After enteric feedings begin, fecal color, odor, and consistency change. Transitional stools usually appear on the second or third day after feedings begin. These stools have a higher water content than meconium.
   C. The formula-fed neonate passes pasty, greenish brown stools with a strong odor.
   D. Stools from the breastfed neonate are golden-yellow, sweet smelling, and more liquid.

19._____

20. The immune system is deficient at birth. Exposure to substances like bacteria activates components of the immune response.
Bacterial infection occurs in about _____ % of neonates; viral infection occurs in about _____ %.

   A. 2; 8   B. 4; 10   C. 6; 12   D. 8; 14

20._____

21. Which of the following statements does NOT provide correct information about the neonate's immune response mechanism?

   A. The various elements of the immune system recognize, remember, respond to, and eliminate foreign substances called antibodies which may invade the body's protective barriers or arise from malignant cell transformation.
   B. When local barriers and inflammation fail to fight off antigenic invasion, the immune system initiates a humoral or cell-mediated response.

21._____

C. The cell-mediated response is carried out by the mononuclear phagocytic system, which includes cells in the thymus, lymphoid tissue, liver, spleen, and bone marrow.
D. Cells involved in the immune response include lymphocytes, specifically T cells and B cells, granulocytes, monocytes, red blood cells, and platelets.

22. Humoral immunity in neonates is MOST important against

    A. bacterial reinfection
    B. viral reinfection
    C. reinfection by group B streptococci and staphylococci
    D. all of the above

23. All of the following are true about fetal and/or neonatal immunoglobulin G (IgG) EXCEPT:

    A. IgG is the most abundant immunoglobulin and is synthesized in response to bacteria, viruses, and fungal organisms. Fetal IgG appears by the twelfth week of gestation, with levels increasing significantly during the last trimester.
    B. IgG is active against gram-positive cocci, some viruses, meningococci, H. influenzae, and diphtheria and tetanus toxins if the mother has been exposed to these agents.
    C. The neonate has protection against most childhood diseases, including diphtheria, measles, and smallpox, provided the mother has antibodies to these diseases. Since IgG does not act against gram-negative rods, such as Escherichia coli and Enterobacter, the neonate is more susceptible to infection by these agents.
    D. By age 6 months, maternally acquired IgG is depleted. By then, however, the body usually produces enough IgG to replace the lost antibodies.

24. Which of the following is NOT true about fetal and/or neonatal immunoglobulin M (IgM)?

    A. IgM is the first immunoglobulin produced by antigenic challenge and is the major antibody in blood type incompatibilities and gram-negative bacterial infections.
    B. Maternal IgM does not cross the placenta; however, by the 20th week of gestation, the fetus produces IgM in response to antigenic exposure.
    C. IgM provides a long-lasting or permanent active immunity resulting from antigenic stimulation through inoculation or natural immunity.
    D. Low IgM levels in the neonate may signal perinatal infection.

25. Studies about fetal and/or neonatal immunoglobulin A (IgA) do NOT claim that

    A. IgA appears in all body secretions and is considered to be the major antibody in the mucosal linings of the intestines and bronchi
    B. maternal IgA is transferred to the fetus via the placenta. Fetal IgA appears by the 16th week of gestation.
    C. combining with a mucosal protein, IgA is secreted onto mucosal surfaces as a secretory antibody also called secretory IgA
    D. Secretory IgA, which is present in breast milk, confers some passive immunity on the breastfed infant. Secretory IgA also limits bacterial growth in the GI tract.

KEY (CORRECT ANSWERS)

1.	C	11.	C
2.	C	12.	D
3.	D	13.	A
4.	C	14.	A
5.	B	15.	C
6.	A	16.	B
7.	A	17.	D
8.	D	18.	C
9.	B	19.	C
10.	C	20.	A

21. A
22. D
23. D
24. D
25. B

TEST 3

DIRECTIONS: Each question or incomplete statement is followed by several suggested answers or completions. Select the one that BEST answers the question or completes the statement. *PRINT THE LETTER OF THE CORRECT ANSWER IN THE SPACE AT THE RIGHT.*

1. Which of the following is NOT correct about the mechanism of cell-mediated immunity? 1.___

    A. This immune response is most apparent in localized inflammations triggered by fungi, viruses, tumors, and organ transplants.
    B. Recognizing a foreign antigen, T cells mobilize tissue macrophages in the presence of migration inhibitory factor.
    C. The substance mentioned in para B triggers chemical reactions that convert local macrophages into phagocytes and prevent macrophages from leaving the invasion site until they have destroyed the antigen.
    D. The breastfed infant may acquire passive immunity to diseases such as polio, mumps, influenza, and chicken pox through the cell-mediated response.

2. The viral and nonviral agents that cause congenital infections are collectively called *TORCH,* which is an acronym for 2.___

    A. tuberculosis, others, reovirus, CMV, and herpes
    B. trypanosomiasis, others, rubella, CMV, and hepatitis
    C. toxoplasmosis, others, rubella, CMV, and herpes
    D. tuberculosis, orbivirus, rubeola, CMV, and hepatitis

3. Congenital bacterial infections may arise from bacterial organisms that travel to the fetus through the placenta. The one of the following organisms that does NOT cause such infections is 3.___

    A. listeria monocytogenes B. E. coli and klebsiella
    C. streptococcus pneumoniae D. herpes simplex

4. All of the following are known to be routes of congenital bacterial infections EXCEPT 4.___

    A. mother's cervix, amniotic membrane
    B. fetal skin and mucus membranes
    C. intervillous placental spaces, umbilical cord to the fetal circulation
    D. respiratory airways via aspiration

5. All of the following are true about the neonate's neurologic system EXCEPT: 5.___

    A. The neonate's neurologic function is controlled primarily by the brain stem and spinal cord. The autonomic nervous system and brain stem coordinate respiratory and cardiac functions.
    B. All cranial nerves are present at birth fully sheathed with myelin, a substance essential for smooth nerve impulse transmission.
    C. At birth, the brain measures about one-fourth the size of the adult brain. The brain grows and matures in a cephalocaudal direction.
    D. The brain needs a constant supply of glucose for energy and a relatively high oxygen level to maintain adequate cellular metabolism, thus preventing complications such as impaired gas exchange and hypoglycemia.

6. Which of the following statements is NOT correct about the neonate's nerve tract development?

    A. Sensory, cerebellar, and extrapyramidal nerve pathways are the first to develop, which accounts for the neonate's strong senses of hearing, taste, and smell.
    B. The cerebellum governs gross voluntary movement and helps maintain equilibrium.
    C. The extrapyramidal tract controls reflexive gross motor movement and postural adjustment by regulating reciprocal flexion and extension of muscle groups, thus maintaining smooth, coordinated movement.
    D. The neonate's nerve tract development is completed by the 30th week of gestation.

7. At birth, the endocrine system is anatomically mature but functionally immature. Complex interactions between the neurologic and endocrine systems help coordinate adaptation to extrauterine life.
   Such interactions take place along the _____ major feedback pathway.

    A. parasympathetic-adrenal medulla
    B. hypothalamic-anterior pituitary
    C. hypothalamic-posterior pituitary
    D. all of the above

8. The posterior pituitary gland secretes only a limited amount of a hormone which limits urine production. Insufficient amounts of this hormone contribute to the neonatal increased risk of dehydration.
   What hormone is this?

    A. Gonadotropin-releasing hormone (GnRH)
    B. Follicle-stimulating hormone (FSH)
    C. Luteinizing hormone (LH)
    D. Antidiuretic hormone (ADH)

9. Which of the following statements is NOT correct about the metabolic changes in the neonate?

    A. At birth, the neonate's serum glucose level usually measures 60% to 70% of the maternal serum glucose level. Over the next 2 hours, this level falls, stabilizing between 35 and 40 mg/dl.
    B. By 6 hours after birth, the neonate's serum glucose level usually rises to about 60 mg/dl, unless the neonate experiences cold stress, delayed feeding, metabolic abnormalities, or sepsis.
    C. The serum calcium level decreases at birth but usually stabilizes between 24 and 48 hours after birth. A level below 12 mg/dl reflects hypocalcemia.
    D. Most commonly, hypocalcemia arises within the first 2 days or at 6 to 10 days after birth. Hypocalcemia may result from hypoxemia, interrupted maternal calcium transfer, or infant formula with an improper calcium-to-phosphorus ratio, which needs to be 2:1 to be normal.

10. Initially, the full-term neonate's core temperature falls by approximately 0.54F per minute. Thus, under normal delivery conditions, it may drop _____ °F before the neonate leaves the delivery room.

    A. 4.4   B. 5.4   C. 6.4   D. 7.4

11. Which of the following statements provides CORRECT information about Neutral Thermal Environment (NTE)?

    A. For an unclothed, full-term neonate on the first day after birth, NTE ranges from 89.6° F to 93.2° F. Within this temperature range, oxygen consumption and carbon dioxide production are lowest and core temperature is normal.
    B. To maintain body temperature within the NTE, the neonate makes vasomotor adjustments, i.e., vasocon-striction to conserve heat and vasodilation to release heat.
    C. Environmental temperatures below or above the NTE increase oxygen consumption and boost the metabolic rate, i.e., the amount of energy expended over a given unit of time.
    D. All of the above

12. All of the following characteristics place the neonate at a physiologic disadvantage for thermoregulation, increasing the risk of hypothermia EXCEPT

    A. a small body surface relative to mass
    B. limited subcutaneous fat deposition to provide insulation
    C. vasomotor instability
    D. limited metabolic capacity

13. Heat loss, which begins at delivery, CANNOT occur through

    A. radiation
    B. conduction
    C. evaporation
    D. conversion

14. Which of the following statements is NOT true concerning the mechanisms of heat loss in the neonate?

    A. Evaporation occurs when fluids, such as insensible water, visible perspiration, and pulmonary fluids, turn to vapor in dry air. The drier the environment, the greater the evaporative heat loss.
    B. Conduction takes place when the neonate's skin directly contacts a cooler object, e.g., a cold bed or scale; therefore, any metal surface on which the neonate will be placed should be padded.
    C. A cooler solid surface not in direct contact with the neonate can cause heat loss through radiation. Common sources of radiant heat loss include incubator walls and windows.
    D. Heat loss from the body surface to cooler surrounding air occurs through conversion. It increases in drafty environments. Thus, a delivery room cooled for the comfort of personnel may cause significant conversive heat loss in the neonate.

15. In a cold environment or in other stressful circumstances, the neonate defends against heat lost through all of the following EXCEPT

    A. vasomotor control
    B. thermal insulation, muscle activity
    C. shivering thermogenesis
    D. nonshivering thermogenesis

16. Which of the following statements does NOT correctly explain nonshivering thermogenesis?

    A. Defined as the production of heat through lipolysis of brown fat, nonshivering thermogenesis is the neonate's most efficient heat production mechanism because it increases the metabolic rate minimally.
    B. Brown fat, which is a type of adipose tissue and is named for its brown color due to its rich vascular supply, dense cellular content, and numerous nerve endings, accounts for up to 3% of a full-term neonate's total weight.
    C. Brown fat is deposited around the neck, head, heart, great vessels, kidneys, and adrenal glands; between the scapula; behind the sternum; and in the axillae.
    D. The brain, liver, and skeletal muscles take part in nonshivering thermogenesis. In response to heat loss, sympathetic nerves stimulate the release of norepinephrine, the major mediator of the mechanism. Norepinephrine stimulates oxidation of brown fat, causing increased heat production.

17. All of the following are correct about the fetal and/or neonatal integumentary system EXCEPT:

    A. The healthy neonate is moist and warm to the touch and may have fine, downy hair called lanugo over the shoulders and back.
    B. The neonate's skin serves as the first line of defense against infection. The outermost skin layer, the stratum corneum, is fused with the vernix caseosa, which is a greasy white substance produced by sebaceous glands. The vernix caseosa coats the fetal skin and protects it from the amniotic fluid.
    C. The full-term neonate's skin appears erythematous for several minutes after birth but soon takes on a normal color.
    D. In many neonates, vasomotor instability, capillary stasis, and high hemoglobin levels lead to acrocyano-sis, characterized by bluish discoloration of the hands and feet. Skin color and circulation usually improve with warming of the hands and feet.

18. All of the following correctly describe the neonatal reproductive system EXCEPT:

    A. The reproductive system is anatomically and functionally immature at birth; however, the female's ovaries contain all potential ova, which decrease in number from birth to maturity by roughly 90%.
    B. In approximately 90% of males, the testes have descended into the scrotum by birth, although no sperm appear until puberty.
    C. High maternal estrogen levels may cause transient side effects in the neonate, e.g., breast hypertrophy with or without witch's milk may appear in both male and female neonates.
    D. The female may have pseudomenstruation, a mucoid or blood-tinged vaginal discharge caused by the sudden increase in hormone levels after birth.

19. Which of the following statements about the neonatal visual capacities is NOT correct?

    A. The neonate's visual acuity is limited to a distance of approximately 9" to 12". Black and white images hold the neonate's gaze longer than color images.
    B. The neonate can conjugate the eyes at or just after birth; however, immature neuromuscular control limits visual accommodation for the first 2 weeks after birth.
    C. Immature neuromuscular control sometimes causes transient strabismus. Also, the epicanthal fold covering the inner canthus of the eyes may narrow the visible width of the sclera beside the iris, giving a neonate the appearance of having crossed eyes, called pseudostrabismus.

D. An adult-level visual acuity is achieved by age 6 months, which may improve even more rapidly in the neonate exposed to various pleasing objects in a range of colors, shapes, and contrasts.

20. Which of the following statements is CORRECT about neonatal hearing capacities?

    A. The neonate can hear at birth. In fact, hearing begins even earlier; the fetus can hear extrauterine sounds as well as noises originating in maternal body systems, including variable low-pitched sounds in the maternal cardiovascular and GI systems.
    B. Hearing is well-established after aeration of the eustachian tube and drainage of blood, vernix caseosa, amniotic fluid, and mucus from the outer ear.
    C. Able to differentiate sounds on the basis of frequency, intensity, and pattern, the neonate responds more readily to sounds below 4,000 Hz.
    D. All of the above

21. All of the following statements about neonatal sensory capacities are correct EXCEPT:

    A. The neonate has well-developed tactile perception, which serves as a stimulus for the first breath. The most sensitive body areas include the face, hands, and soles.
    B. The neonate differentiates among tastes by the first or second day after birth.
    C. Physiologic changes associated with pain include increased pulse and decreased blood pressure during and after a painful procedure.
    D. Sensitivity to olfactory stimuli increases over the first 4 days after birth.

22. The neonate's initial hours are characterized by a predictable, identifiable series of behavioral and physiologic characteristics which were collectively described by Desmond and Associates as the *periods of neonatal reactivity.*
    All of the following provide correct information about the periods of neonatal reactivity EXCEPT:

    A. *First period of reactivity,* beginning just after birth, lasts roughly 60 minutes. The neonate has a strong desire to suckle during this period, so breastfeeding may be initiated. Neonatal adaptations during this period are regulated mainly by the sympathetic nervous system. Visible features of this period include spontaneous startles, the Moro reflex, grimacing, sucking motions, sudden cries that stop abruptly, fine tremors of the jaw or extremities, blinking, and jerking eye movements. Also, irregular respirations, tachypnea, and nasal flaring unrelated to respiratory distress may occur.
    B. In *sleep stage,* the neonate typically falls asleep about 2 to 3 hours after birth and remains asleep from a few minutes to 2 to 4 hours. While asleep, the neonate's respiratory rate increases while the heart rate ranges from 120 to 140 beats/minute.
    C. In *second period of reactivity,* which begins when the neonate awakens after the sleep stage, the heart rate is labile and episodes of bradycardia and tachycardia occur. Thick oral secretions frequently cause gagging and emesis. The respiratory rate, ranging from about 30 to 60 breaths/minute, is irregular and may include brief apneic pauses and periodic tachyp-nea. The neonate usually expels meconium from the GI tract during this period.
    D. The second period of reactivity lasts from 12 to 18 hours, and as it ends, the neonate becomes more stable and the respiratory and cardiac rates normalize.

23. The sleep and awake states encompass the behavioral states used in the Brazelton Neonatal Behavioral Assessment Scale (BNBAS). Developed by Brazelton to measure a neonate's capabilities, the BNBAS assesses neonatal behavioral responses and elicited responses as well as behavioral states.
Brazelton classified the neonate's state of consciousness into six states, dividing them further into _____ sleep state(s) and _____ awake states.

    A. one; five
    B. two; four
    C. three; three
    D. four; two

24. All of the following statements provide appropriate information about sleep states EXCEPT:

    A. In *deep sleep* state, except for occasional startle reflexes, no spontaneous activity occurs. Respirations are even and regular.
    B. In *deep sleep* state, the neonate cannot be aroused by external stimuli with the exception of breastfeeding, due to strong mother-infant bonding.
    C. In *light sleep* state, the neonate's eyes are closed and rapid eye movements (REM's) occur. External stimuli may arouse the neonate in this state.
    D. Variable breathing patterns, random movements, and sucking motions typify light sleep.

25. Which of the following statements is NOT correct about one of the awake states of the neonate?

    A. In *drowsy state,* the neonate's eyes are closed but the eyelids may flutter frequently. Muscle movements are smooth, with intermittent spontaneous activity and startles.
    B. In *alert state,* the neonate's eyes are open, bright, and shining, and the neonate focuses on the source of stimulation. Also, the neonate makes purposeful movements and shows good eye-hand coordination. This state is considered the optimal state of arousal, ideal for parent-neonate contact or breastfeeding initiation.
    C. In *active state,* the neonate's movements increase compared to alert state, and external stimuli cause eye and body movements.
    D. In *crying state,* the neonate responds to both internal and external stimuli. The neonate in the crying state typically progresses to increased motor activity, with thrusting movements of the extremities and spontaneous startles.

KEY (CORRECT ANSWERS)

1. A
2. C
3. D
4. A
5. B

6. D
7. D
8. D
9. C
10. B

11. D
12. A
13. D
14. D
15. C

16. B
17. C
18. D
19. B
20. D

21. C
22. D
23. B
24. B
25. A

EXAMINATION SECTION
TEST 1

DIRECTIONS: Each question or incomplete statement is followed by several suggested answers or completions. Select the one that BEST answers the question or completes the statement. *PRINT THE LETTER OF THE CORRECT ANSWER IN THE SPACE AT THE RIGHT.*

1. All of the following are correct about neonatal assessment proceedings EXCEPT: 1.____
    A. Neonatal assessment proceeds from an immediate determination of the Apgar score to a complete physical assessment. Determination of the Apgar score takes place in the delivery area.
    B. The Apgar scoring system is used to estimate the severity of respiratory and neurologic depression at birth by rating certain physical signs.
    C. Within 24 to 48 hours after birth, the nurse should conduct a complete physical assessment to determine how well the neonate is adapting to the extrauterine environment and to check for obvious problems and major anomalies.
    D. After the physical assessment, the nurse estimates the neonatal gestational age and, if necessary, conducts a formal gestational-age assessment, using a special assessment tool, to determine gestational age precisely.

2. Determination of preterm or postterm status is usually established by the time of delivery. 2.____
The risk of preterm delivery does NOT increase with
    A. various intrapartal factors, such as multiple gestation, fetal infection, preeclampsia, premature rupture of the membranes, abruptio placentae, hydramnios, placenta previa, and poor prenatal care
    B. maternal history of abdominal surgery, uterine anomalies, trauma, cervical incompetency, infection, or previous preterm delivery
    C. chronic maternal disease, such as cardiovascular disease, renal disease, or diabetes mellitus
    D. maternal age under 22

3. With a postterm neonate, the intrapartal history may include 3.____
    A. weight loss
    B. reduced uterine size
    C. decreased abdominal circumference
    D. all of the above

4. The prenatal and intrapartal history may suggest a birth-weight variation. Such variations 4.____
include *small for gestational age (SGA),* which is defined as a birth weight that falls below the tenth percentile for gestational age on the Colorado intrauterine growth chart. Risk factors for delivery of an SGA neonate include all of the following EXCEPT
    A. low socioeconomic status, long stature
    B. age under 19 or over 34
    C. low prepregnancy weight, multiparity
    D. previous delivery of an SGA neonate

5. Which of the following statements about the term large for *gestational age (LGA)* is NOT correct?
   A. LGA is defined as a birth weight that exceeds the ninetieth percentile for gestational age on the Colorado intrauterine growth chart.
   B. Typically, the diagnosis of LGA is established during the antepartal period, when fundal height appears disproportionate to gestational weeks.
   C. Since diabetes mellitus is a leading cause of accelerated intrauterine growth, an elevated maternal serum glucose level may result in an LGA fetus.
   D. Women identified as high risk by history or clinical assessment deliver about two-thirds of LGA neonates.

6. Features to assess in the general survey include all of the following EXCEPT
   A. respiratory and heart rates
   B. posture and head size
   C. lanugo and vernix caseosa
   D. cry and state of alertness

7. After assessing general appearance, the nurse measures vital signs. Which of the following would NOT be included?
   A. Temperature
   B. Respiratory rate
   C. Blood pressure
   D. Heart rhythm

8. The neonate's anthropometric measurements include all of the following EXCEPT
   A. weight
   B. crown-to-heel length
   C. head and chest circumferences
   D. head-to-heel length

9. The average full-term gestation lasts about _____ weeks from _____.
   A. 32; fertilization
   B. 42; the first day of the last menstrual period
   C. 36; fertilization
   D. 40; the first day of the last menstrual period

10. Which of the following statements gives CORRECT information about recording the vital signs of the neonate?
    A. The nurse should measure the neonate's vital signs every 15 minutes for the first hour after birth.
    B. If the signs remain stable for the first hour after birth, the nurse should measure them at least every hour for the next 6 hours.
    C. If the signs remain stable for the 7 hours alter birth, the nurse should measure them at least every 8 hours until discharge,
    D. All of the above

11. When measuring the axillary temperature of the neonate, the nurse should place the thermometer in the axilla and hold it along the outer aspect of the neonate's chest, between the axillary line and the arm, for at least _____ minute(s).
    A. 1   B. 2   C. 3   D. 4

12. To evaluate breath sounds, the nurse should auscultate both the neonate's anterior and posterior lung fields, placing the stethoscope over each lung lobe for AT LEAST _____ seconds for a total time of _____ minute(s).
    A. 20; 3   B. 15; 2   C. 10; 1 1/2   D. 5; 1

13. To assess the neonate's pulse, place the stethoscope over the apical impulse on the _____ intercostal space at the _____ midclavicular line over the cardiac apex and listen for 1 minute.
    A. second to third; right
    B. fourth to fifth; left
    C. sixth to seventh; right
    D. eighth to ninth; left

14. Which of the following is NOT a correct measure for taking the neonate's blood pressure?
    A. When using a Doppler probe, place the cuff directly over the brachial or popliteal artery to ensure an accurate reading.
    B. For the most accurate reading, keep the cuffed arm or leg extended during cuff inflation.
    C. Make sure to choose the correct cuff size, since improper size may cause a misleading reading. Cuff width should be double the circumference of the neonate's arm.
    D. Place the cuff one or two fingerbreadths above the antecubital or popliteal area. With the stethoscope held directly over the chosen artery, hold the cuffed extremity firmly to keep it extended, then inflate the cuff.

15. All of the following statements are correct regarding the neonate's gestational age assessment EXCEPT:
    A. Gestational age should be assessed for any neonate who has a suspected alteration in the intrauterine growth pattern or weighs less than 2,000 gm.
    B. The most common gestational-age assessment tools are the Dubowitz tool and the Ballard tool.
    C. The Dubowitz tool includes 11 external and 10 neurologic signs.
    D. The Ballard tool consists of 7 physical maturity and 6 neuromuscular maturity criteria.

16. Of the following physical assessment findings, the one NOT considered normal for the neonate is:
    A. 120 to 160 heart beats/minute with regular rhythm and no audible heart murmur, except for slight murmur heard over base or left sternal border until foramen ovale closes. Thrill is absent except for first few hours after birth.
    B. The average head circumference is 32 to 35 cm. The anterior fontanel is diamond-shaped, measures 2x3x5 cm. and normally closes by age 18 months. The posterior fontanel is triangular-shaped, measures 1x1x1 cm. and normally closes by age 2 months.
    C. Eyes are spaced 3.5 cm. apart. Positive doll's eye reflex. Positive sucking, swallowing, rooting, and gag reflexes. Neck has full range of motion, i.e., head can turn to each side equally. Strong and bilaterally equal brachial and radial pulses.
    D. Chest circumference is 30 to 33 cm. Two to four bowel sounds per minute. Enlarged clitoris from maternal hormonal influence. Penis is straight, 2.8 to 4.3 cm long. Testes are descended on at least one side. Strong and bilaterally regular femoral pulses. Symmetrical plantar and patellar reflexes are present.

17. The typical neonate sleeps _____ hours daily, with deep sleep accounting for only about _____ hours of total sleep.
    A. 6 to 16; 8
    B. 8 to 18; 6
    C. 10 to 20; 4
    D. 6 to 20; 6

18. All of the following are true categories of neonatal behavioral responses EXCEPT
    A. habituation and orientation
    B. psychological behaviors
    C. self-quieting ability
    D. variations and motor maturity

19. If habituation does not occur after three presentations of a stimulus, the neonate may be hyperresponsive to external stimuli. A slowed or diminished response from the outset of the first presentation, except during deep sleep, suggests lethargy or hyperresponsiveness.
    Habituation should be tested during the _____ state.
    A. deep sleep
    B. light sleep
    C. drowsy
    D. all of the above

20. All of the following are correct about the Apgar scoring system EXCEPT:
    A. According to this system, every neonate should be rated at exactly 1 and 5 minutes after birth. The maximum score of 10 is rare; the lower the score, the more severely depressed the neonate. A score of 5 or lower indicates severe depression.
    B. Low scores, particularly at 5 minutes, are more likely to predict residual neurologic damage or neonatal death, although most neonates with low 5 minute Apgar scores survive and are normal.
    C. Low Apgar scores may be caused by either perinatal asphyxia or respiratory and neurologic depression from transplacental passage of anesthetics given to the mother.
    D. The neonate with low Apgar scores due to perinatal asphyxia will appear cyanotic or pale and have an increased heart rate and high blood pressure, while a neonate depressed by anesthetics is likely to have normal color, heart rate, and blood pressure at birth.

21. The assessment findings for indications of neonatal distress do NOT include
    A. abdominal distension and bile-stained emesis
    B. frequent apneic episodes and meconium-stained skin
    C. temperature instability and jaundice
    D. persistent, pronounced decrease in heart and respiratory rates from baseline vital signs

22. Which of the following is NOT considered a correct nursing diagnosis for the normal neonate?
    A. Altered patterns of urinary elimination related to inability to maintain fluid balance or renal immaturity
    B. Constipation related to GI immaturity
    C. Diarrhea related to digestive enzyme imbalance
    D. Fluid volume excess related to renal immaturity

23. All of the following are appropriate nursing diagnoses for the normal neonate EXCEPT
    A. hypothermia related to cold stress
    B. potential altered body temperature related to radiant, conductive, convective, or evaporative heat loss or gain
    C. potential for trauma related to decreased vitamin K levels
    D. ineffective airway clearance related to the absence of mucus

24. When caring for the normal neonate, the nurse may have to administer prophylactic vitamin K or other medications by I.M. injection.
    In most cases, the BEST needle size to use to allow medication to reach the muscle without causing excessive pain or trauma is _____-gauge.
    A. 25   B. 22   C. 18   D. 14

25. The nurse should NOT give an injection in the buttocks of the neonate because the
    A. muscle mass here is not well-developed
    B. needle or medication can enter a major vessel
    C. needle or medication can enter a major nerve more easily
    D. all of the above

26. To maintain hydration, the term neonate requires a fluid intake of _____ ml/kg/day.
    A. 100 to 120
    B. 120 to 140
    C. 140 to 160
    D. 160 to 180

27. In the normal neonate, urine output should measure _____ ml/kg/hour
    A. 1 to 2   B. 3 to 4   C. 5 to 6   D. 7 to 8

28. Projectile vomiting or bile-colored emesis in the neonate indicates
    A. esophageal atresia
    B. pyloric stenosis
    C. gastroesophageal reflex (GER)
    D. gastrointestinal blockage

29. The neonate's failure to void within 48 hours may indicate all of the following EXCEPT
    A. inadequate fluid intake
    B. hepatic disorder
    C. fluid retention causing edema
    D. increased water loss

30. Neonatal ophthalmia, an eye infection caused by Neisseria gonorrhea or Chlamydia trachomatis, can be prevented by application of _____ to the eyes shortly after delivery.
    A. 1% silver nitrate solution
    B. 1% tetracycline ointment
    C. 0.5% erythromycin ointment
    D. all of the above

KEY (CORRECT ANSWERS)

1. C	11. C	21. D
2. D	12. D	22. C
3. D	13. B	23. D
4. A	14. C	24. A
5. D	15. A	25. D
6. A	16. C	26. C
7. D	17. C	27. A
8. B	18. B	28. D
9. D	19. D	29. B
10. D	20. D	30. D

TEST 2

DIRECTIONS: Each question or incomplete statement is followed by several suggested answers or completions. Select the one that BEST answers the question or completes the statement. *PRINT THE LETTER OF THE CORRECT ANSWER IN THE SPACE AT THE RIGHT.*

1. Without sufficient vitamin K, the liver cannot synthesize coagulation factors II, VII, IX, and X. This deficiency predisposes the neonate to hemorrhage.
   Thus, the American Academy of Pediatrics recommends a prophylactic I.M. injection of vitamin K1 (phytonadione) of _____ mg. within _____ hour(s) after birth.
   A. 0.5 to 1; one
   B. 1 to 1.5; two
   C. 1.5 to 2; three
   D. 2 to 2.5; four
   1._____

2. All of the following are correct about the circumcision procedure in the neonate EXCEPT:
   A. The main advantage of circumcision is hygienic. The circumcised penis is easier to keep clean and free of smegma, a sebaceous secretion that accumulates under foreskin.
   B. Because the neonate's tight skin makes foreskin retraction difficult, bacterial growth is less common with a circumcised penis.
   C. The major disadvantage of circumcision is the pain and discomfort it causes, and the neonate has a disturbed sleep-awake pattern. To reduce pain, the neonate is given a topical antibiotic.
   D. Petroleum gauze is applied over the penis to prevent bleeding and encrustation and to serve as a protective layer against abrasion from the diaper. The gauze is necessary for only 2 to 3 days after the procedure.
   2._____

3. Of the following examples, the one that does NOT illustrate an appropriate evaluation for the NORMAL neonate is: The neonate
   A. did not appear cyanotic or dusky
   B. maintained a stable body temperature of 96° F to 97.7° F
   C. voided clear amber urine six times in 24 hours
   D. passed a meconium stool 48 hours after birth
   3._____

4. Thorough documentation of all steps of the nursing process not only allows the nurse to evaluate the effectiveness of the care plan, but it also makes the data available to other members of the health care team, helping to ensure consistency of care.
   Documentation for the normal neonate should include all of the following EXCEPT
   A. vital signs, capillary refill time, general appearance
   B. size and shape of fontanels, umbilical cord description
   C. any abnormal physical or behavioral findings, parent teaching
   D. stool and urine passage, strength and symmetry of peripheral nerves
   4._____

5. The physician may order various laboratory tests to check for such neonatal complications as infection, hematologic problems, and metabolic disorders. Of the following, the ABNORMAL laboratory vale is
   A. hematocrit 51% to 56%; hemoglobin 16.5 g/dl
   B. platelets 150,000 to 400,000/mm^3; calcium 7 to 10 mg/dl
   C. serum glucose 40 to 80 mg/dl; total protein 4 to 7 g/dl
   D. WBC total 18,000/mm3; potassium 15 to 20 mEq/liter
   5._____

6. All of the following are considered basic nutrients that supply the body's caloric needs EXCEPT
    A. vitamins and minerals
    B. carbohydrates
    C. proteins
    D. fats

7. The body's MAIN source of calories is
    A. vitamins and minerals
    B. carbohydrates
    C. proteins
    D. fats

8. Concerning the neonate's calories supplied by the basic nutrients, it is TRUE that _____ contain _____ calories per gram and provide _____ % of the neonate's total calories.
    A. carbohydrates; 4; 35 to 55
    B. fats; 9; 30 to 55
    C. proteins; 4; 34.5 to 55
    D. all of the above

9. Vitamins regulate metabolic processes and promote growth and maintenance of body tissue.
    All of the following are fat-soluble vitamins, which can be stored in the body to some extent and normally are not excreted, EXCEPT
    A. A
    B. C
    C. D
    D. K

10. Vitamin B _____ is NOT a water-soluble vitamin.
    A. 2
    B. 3
    C. 6
    D. 12

11. All major minerals and most trace minerals are essential for all of the following body functions EXCEPT
    A. regulation of enzyme metabolism
    B. acid-base balance
    C. nerve and muscle integrity
    D. strengthening of vessel walls

12. _____ is NOT among the major solutes in the neonate's body system.
    A. Calcium
    B. Sodium
    C. Potassium
    D. Urea

13. The major nutritional assessment indices in the infant include all of the following EXCEPT
    A. weight
    B. length
    C. chest circumference
    D. head circumference

14. Under the influence of human placental lactogen, a hormone secreted by the placenta, lactogenesis begins
    A. during the third trimester of pregnancy
    B. during the onset of uteral contractions
    C. as soon as the neonate is delivered under normal circumstances
    D. during the first hour after delivery

15. After delivery of the placenta and the resultant decrease in circulating estrogen and progesterone, the anterior pituitary gland releases a hormone that stimulates mammary gland growth and development.
    This hormone is called
    A. dopamine
    B. enkephalin
    C. endorphin
    D. prolactin

16. In the early days of breastfeeding, restricted sucking time may establish a negative feed- system that can lead to _____ milk production.
    A. excessive
    B. insufficient
    C. no
    D. all of the above

17. The breasts may contain colostrum for up to _____ hours
    A. 24
    B. 48
    C. 72
    D. 96

18. Colostrum contains all of the following contents which function as antibodies EXCEPT
    A. high concentrations of protein
    B. fat-soluble vitamins; minerals
    C. most of the essential fatty acids
    D. immunoglobulins

19. A breastfed infant typically needs to be fed every _____ hours
    A. 1 to 2
    B. 2 to 3
    C. 3 to 4
    D. 4 to 5

20. The amount and frequency of formula feedings vary with infant size, maturity, and activity level
    Daily formula intake averages _____ ml/kg.
    A. 140
    B. 180
    C. 220
    D. 260

21. All of the following are appropriate recommended formula volume and feeding frequencies for infants receiving commercial formula exclusively EXCEPT _____ daily feedings at a volume of _____ ml per feeding for an infant of month(s) of age.
    A. 8; 126; 1
    B. 5; 168; 4
    C. 5; 131; 7 to 9
    D. 4; 141; 12

22. For the client in the antepartal period who will be using infant formula, the nurse should assess for
    A. knowledge of proper feeding techniques
    B. understanding of types of formula
    C. previous experience with infant formula
    D. all of the above

23. Infant factors to assess for include all of the following EXCEPT
    A. excessive drooling, coughing, gagging, or respiratory distress during feeding
    B. amount of formula the infant takes; regurgitation after feeding
    C. signs of glucose intolerance
    D. mucus in regurgitated matter; how readily the infant burps

24. All of the following are appropriate potential nursing diagnoses for problems and etiologies that a nurse may encounter when caring for a client as she begins to nourish her neonate EXCEPT
    A. altered family processes related to both infant feeding and breastfeeding
    B. altered parenting related to infant prematurity and the mother's wish to breastfeed
    C. potential fluid volume deficit related to breastfeeding
    D. body image disturbance related to physiologic changes secondary to formula feeding

25. Of the following, the one which is NOT an appropriate breastfeeding position is the
    A. cradle position
    B. side-lying position
    C. upright position
    D. football hold

26. The nurse should tell the client to expect to breastfeed every _____ hours during the day and _____ hours at night.
    A. 1 to 2; 2 to 3
    B. 2 to 3; 4 to 5
    C. 3 to 4; 5 to 6
    D. 4 to 5; 6 to 7

27. Growth spurts occur at all of the following ages EXCEPT
    A. 10 to 14 days
    B. 6 weeks
    C. 3 to 4 months
    D. 8 to 9 months

28. In North America, feeding schedules for premature infants typically are based on
    A. infant weight
    B. gestational age
    C. ability to bottle-feed without signs of distress
    D. all of the above

29. All of the following are basic methods used to prepare infant formula EXCEPT the _____ method.
    A. multiple-bottle
    B. terminal
    C. onr-bottle
    D. aseptic

30. Which of the following is NOT considered an appropriate position for burping?
    A. Upright
    B. Side-lying
    C. Across the lap
    D. Upright on the lap

KEY (CORRECT ANSWERS)

1. A	11. D	21. A
2. C	12. A	22. D
3. D	13. C	23. C
4. D	14. A	24. D
5. D	15. D	25. C
6. A	16. B	26. B
7. B	17. D	27. D
8. D	18. C	28. D
9. B	19. B	29. A
10. B	20. B	30. B

EXAMINATION SECTION
TEST 1

DIRECTIONS: Each question or incomplete statement is followed by several suggested answers or completions. Select the one that BEST answers the question or completes the statement. *PRINT THE LETTER OF THE CORRECT ANSWER IN THE SPACE AT THE RIGHT.*

1. Which of these occurrences in a postpartal woman would be MOST indicative of an abnormality?

    A. A chill shortly after delivery
    B. A pulse rate of 60 the morning after delivery
    C. Urinary output of 3,000 ml. on the second day after delivery
    D. An oral temperature of 101° F. (38.3° C.) on the third day after delivery

2. While discussing nutrition with the nurse, a woman who is a primigravida says that she eats an egg for breakfast every day.
   The woman should be informed that the absorption of iron from the egg would be BEST facilitated by the woman's also eating _____ at the same meal.

    A. toast   B. butter
    C. orange juice   D. bacon

Questions 3-8.

DIRECTIONS: Questions 3 through 8 are to be answered on the basis of the following information.

Ms. Judy Lee, 28 years old and gravida I, is attending the antepartal clinic regularly. Ms. Lee is carrying twins. In the 38th week of gestation, she is admitted to the hospital in labor. Her membranes have ruptured.

3. Since Ms. Lee's admission, the nurse has been able to hear and count the heartbeats of both twins. Suppose that at a later time during Ms. Lee's labor, the nurse can hear only one heartbeat, even after several attempts. Which of these interpretations of this finding would be ACCURATE?

    A. Inaudibility of one of the heartbeats can result from a change in the position of the twins, but it could also be due to fetal distress; prompt evaluation of the situation by the physician is mandatory.
    B. Muffled fetal heartbeats are common when uterine contractions are strong and frequent, as they are in a multiple pregnancy; more frequent evaluation of the fetal heartbeats is advisable.
    C. Inability to hear one heartbeat in a twin pregnancy can normally be expected at intervals throughout labor; no action is indicated.
    D. Inability to hear fetal heartbeats in a twin pregnancy does not indicate fetal difficulty unless accompanied by additional symptoms; amniotic fluid should be examined for meconium staining.

4. Ms. Lee's labor progresses, and she delivers spontaneously two girls - one weighs 4 lbs. (1,814 gm.) and the other weighs 4 lb. 8 oz. (2,041 gm.). The twins are transferred to the premature nursery, and Ms. Lee is transferred to the postpartum unit.
Which of these concepts should be MOST basic to planning care for the Lee twins?

   A. Circulatory function is enhanced by frequent change of position.
   B. A well-lubricated skin is resistant to excoriation and damage.
   C. A premature infant's rectal temperature reflects the infant's ability to conserve heat.
   D. Optimal environmental temperature results in minimal oxygen consumption in the premature infant.

5. The method used for a premature infant's first formula feeding and the time at which it is begun will be based CHIEFLY upon the infant's

   A. birth weight
   B. degree of hydration
   C. level of physiologic maturity
   D. total body surface

6. The smaller of the Lee twins is to be gavaged.
In determining the location of the catheter after its insertion into the infant, it would be MOST desirable to insert

   A. the tip of a large syringe into the catheter and withdraw an amount of air equal to the amount of feeding
   B. a few drops of sterile water into the catheter, hold the end of the catheter below the level of the infant's stomach, and observe it for drainage of gastric contents
   C. about 0.5 to 1 ml. of air into the catheter and listen to the infant's abdomen with a stethoscope
   D. about 5 ml. of sterile water into the catheter and observe the infant's respirations

7. On her second postpartum day, Ms. Lee says to the nurse,
I've been to the bathroom four times in the past hour to urinate. The funny thing about it is that I only pass a small amount of urine each time.
Which of these initial actions by the nurse would demonstrate the BEST judgment?

   A. Palpate Ms. Lee's abdomen for bladder distention.
   B. Explain to Ms. Lee that frequent voiding is expected during the first few days after delivery.
   C. Advise Ms. Lee to use a bedpan for her next voiding.
   D. Discuss with Ms. Lee the relationship between trauma during delivery and signs of bladder irritation during the postpartum period.

8. On the third postpartum day, Ms. Lee is discharged. The twins are to remain until they have reached an appropriate weight. When the twins are to be discharged, Mr. and Ms. Lee come to the hospital to take them home.
Which of these statements, if made by Ms. Lee, would indicate the BEST understanding of her babies' needs?

   A. Our babies' needs are different from those of full-term infants, and we will do all we can to protect them.
   B. We are going to try very hard to counteract the effects of our babies' having been born prematurely.

C. For a while the smaller baby will need special attention, and then we will be able to treat both of our babies similarly.
D. We expect to enjoy our babies and will give them the kind of care babies need.

Questions 9-18.

DIRECTIONS: Questions 9 through 18 are to be answered on the basis of the following information.

Ms. Angela Dobbs, 32 years old and gravida I, is now in her third trimester of pregnancy. She has had diabetes mellitus since the age of 16 and has been attending the antepartal clinic regularly for the past 5 months.

9. Compared with Ms. Dobbs' insulin requirements when she was not pregnant, it can be expected that the insulin dosage during her third trimester will

    A. remain the same
    B. be increased
    C. be decreased
    D. be increased or decreased, depending upon fetal activity

10. At 30 weeks' gestation, Ms. Dobbs has an ultrasonic examination. The results of this examination disclose information about the fetus'

    A. circulatory function
    B. gestational age
    C. presence of surfactant
    D. presence of congenital defects

11. Because the incidence of fetal death is higher in women who have diabetes mellitus, indications of placental insufficiency should be suspected if Ms. Dobbs has a(n)

    A. sustained drop in her blood glucose level
    B. urinary output of more than 1500 ml. a day
    C. increase in the secretion of gonadotropin
    D. albumin content in her urine of +1

12. At 35 weeks' gestation, Ms. Dobbs is admitted to the hospital for evaluation of her pregnancy and diabetic status. Ms. Dobbs is to have a urinary estriol level determination. Which of these instructions should be among those given to her about collecting the urine for this procedure? Collect

    A. the first morning specimen before eating breakfast
    B. a specimen about an hour after the evening meal
    C. a twenty-four hour specimen
    D. a clean-voided specimen

13. Ms. Dobbs is to have an amniocentesis done to determine the lecithin/sphingomyelin (L/S) ratio.
    The purpose of this study is to

    A. assess placental functioning
    B. assess the amount of fetal body fat
    C. determine fetal kidney functioning
    D. determine fetal pulmonary maturity

14. Ms. Dobbs has a cesarean section and is delivered of a boy who weighs 8 lb. 4 oz. (3,742 gm.). He is transferred to the intensive care nursery. Ms. Dobbs is transferred to the postpartum unit from the recovery room.
Postpartum orders for Ms. Dobbs include an estrogen preparation to

   A. promote sodium excretion
   B. suppress the production of chorionic gonadotropin
   C. inhibit secretion of the lactogenic hormone
   D. diminish lochial flow

15. Two hours after delivery, the nurse observes that Baby Boy Dobbs is lethargic and has developed mild generalized cyanosis and twitching.
In view of the fact that his mother has diabetes mellitus, the infant is PROBABLY exhibiting symptoms of a

   A. low blood sugar level
   B. high CO_2 level
   C. subnormal temperature
   D. withdrawal from insulin

16. Because Ms. Dobbs has diabetes mellitus, her infant should be assessed for the presence of

   A. a blood group incompatibility
   B. meconium ileus
   C. phenylketonuria
   D. a congenital abnormality

17. Ms. Dobbs is bottle-feeding her baby. Ms. Dobbs, who has previously observed a demonstration of diapering, is changing her baby's diaper for the first time, under the supervision of the registered nurse. Ms. Dobbs is holding the baby's feet correctly, but when she starts to raise his legs to remove the diaper, the feet slip from her grasp, and the baby's legs drop back onto the mattress of the bassinet. The baby whimpers briefly, and Ms. Dobbs looks dismayed.
Which of these responses by the nurse would be BEST?

   A. I'll show you again how to change the baby's diaper, Ms. Dobbs.
   B. I'll diaper the baby for you this time, Ms. Dobbs.
   C. You've almost got it, Ms. Dobbs. Try again?
   D. Why are you so nervous, Ms. Dobbs?

18. Some time after discharge, Ms. Dobbs calls the hospital to report the loss of her baby's birth certificate. Where would it be BEST for her to apply for a duplicate? The

   A. record room of the hospital where the baby was born
   B. agency that records vital statistics for the community in which the baby was born
   C. Census Bureau
   D. National Office of Vital Statistics

Questions 19-25.

DIRECTIONS: Questions 19 through 25 are to be answered on the basis of the following information.

Ms. Linda Young, a 17-year-old high school student, attends the antepartal clinic on a regular basis. This is Linda's first pregnancy.

19. Linda is now 7 months pregnant.
In assessing whether Linda is retaining abnormal amounts of fluid, it would be ESPECIALLY significant that she has gained

   A. 3 lb. (1,361 gm.) during the past week
   B. 4 1/2 lb. (2,041 gm.) since her last clinic visit a month ago
   C. 11 lb. (4,990 gm.) in the second trimester of pregnancy
   D. 14 lb. (6,350 gm.) since the onset of pregnancy

19.____

20. Which of these measures will contribute MOST to the prevention of postpartal uterine infections?

   A. Routine use of serologic tests for syphilis early in the antepartal period
   B. Limitation of sexual intercourse during the last six weeks of pregnancy
   C. Maintenance of cleanliness of the perineal area during labor
   D. Taking showers or sponge baths exclusively during the last six weeks of pregnancy

20.____

21. At term, Linda is admitted to the hospital in active labor. Linda's cervix is 2 cm. dilated and 80% effaced. Which of these interpretations of these findings is CORRECT?
The

   A. cervix is 2 cm. short of complete dilatation, and it is 80% thinner than it was before labor started
   B. cervix is still 2 cm. long, and 80% of the thinning of the cervix is completed
   C. walls of the cervix are 2 cm. thick, and 80% of the widening of the cervical opening has been achieved
   D. opening of the cervix is 2 cm. wide, and the cervical canal is 80% shorter than normal

21.____

22. Linda has an episiotomy and delivers a 7 lb. (3,175 gm.) boy. Baby Boy Young is transferred to the nursery and Linda is transferred to the postpartum unit. Linda plans to bottle-feed her baby. The nurse is assessing Baby Boy Young.
Which of these observations, if made, would be considered characteristics of a newborn?

   A. Branlike desquamation of the hands and fee; alternating limpness and stiffness of the body; and pink, moist skin
   B. Cool, mottled hands and feet; quivering lower jaw; and flexion of body parts
   C. Clenched fists; arching of the back when recumbent; and frequent crying
   D. Butterfly-shaped area of pigmentation at the base of the spine; extension of the arms and legs when the head is turned to the side; and diaphragmatic breathing

22.____

23. When Linda has been admitted to the postpartum unit, she says to the nurse, *I'm so glad my baby is a boy. Maybe Jack will marry me now because he'll be so proud to have a son.*
    It is probably MOST justifiable to say that Linda

    A. wants to get married in order to gain her independence from her family
    B. is capable of subordinating her personal needs to the needs of others
    C. is showing a beginning awareness of the problems associated with having a baby out of wedlock
    D. lacks insight into the factors that contribute to a successful marriage

24. When Baby Boy Young is brought to his mother for the first time to be fed, Linda asks the nurse, *What's wrong with my baby's eyes? He looks cross-eyed.*
    Which of these initial responses by the nurse would probably be MOST helpful?

    A. Babies seem to be cross-eyed for a while after birth because the muscles in their eyes aren't able to work together.
    B. You feel that your baby's eyes are abnormal?
    C. I can see that you're upset about this. It would be advisable for you to talk with the doctor about it.
    D. Your baby will appear cross-eyed for some time because his eyes won't be completely developed until he is about six months old.

25. When Linda is talking with the nurse about feeding her baby, she says, *I've heard that if I breastfed him, he'd develop a close feeling toward me more quickly. I had planned to bottle-feed him.*
    The nurse's initial reply should convey which of these understandings about the development of a mother-child relationship?

    A. A satisfactory mother-child relationship will develop more readily through breast-feeding than bottle-feeding.
    B. Holding the baby during bottle-feeding will help to promote a good mother-child relationship.
    C. The times at which the baby is fed by the mother will affect the quality of the mother-child relationship more than the feeding method.
    D. Since bottle-feeding is less complicated than breastfeeding, the mother will be able to focus more attention on mothering functions such as cuddling and talking while the baby is eating.

KEY (CORRECT ANSWERS)

1. D
2. C
3. A
4. D
5. C

6. C
7. A
8. D
9. B
10. B

11. A
12. C
13. D
14. C
15. A

16. D
17. C
18. B
19. A
20. C

21. D
22. B
23. D
24. A
25. B

TEST 2

DIRECTIONS: Each question or incomplete statement is followed by several suggested answers or completions. Select the one that BEST answers the question or completes the statement. *PRINT THE LETTER OF THE CORRECT ANSWER IN THE SPACE AT THE RIGHT.*

1. The instructions that are ESPECIALLY important to give to a pregnant woman who has heart disease are:

    A. Increase protein intake
    B. Take no drugs unless they have been prescribed
    C. Limit high-calorie foods
    D. Avoid fatigue

1.____

Questions 2-9.

DIRECTIONS: Questions 2 through 9 are to be answered on the basis of the following information.

Ms. Mary White, 35 years old, is pregnant for the third time. She is receiving antepartal care from a private physician. Ms. White is in the seventh month of pregnancy and has symptoms of preeclampsia.

2. The physician instructs Ms. White not to eat foods which have a high sodium content. The nurse tells Ms. White about foods containing sodium and then asks her to identify foods lowest in sodium.
Which of these foods, if selected by Ms. White, would be CORRECT?

    A. Creamed chipped beef on dry toast
    B. Cheese sandwich on whole wheat toast
    C. Frankfurter on a roll
    D. Tomato stuffed with diced chicken

2.____

3. In Ms. White's 39th week of gestation, her physician recommends that she be hospitalized. When the physician leaves after examining Ms. White, Ms. White says to the nurse, *It's easy for you people to say, "Go to the hospital," but it's not so easy for me to do it. I can't go just like that!*
After acknowledging her feeling, which of these approaches by the nurse would probably be BEST?

    A. Stress to Ms. White that her husband would want her to do what is best for her health.
    B. Explore with Ms. White ways that immediate hospitali-zation could be arranged.
    C. Repeat the physician's reasons for advising immediate hospitalization for Ms. White.
    D. Explain to Ms. White that she is ultimately responsible for her own welfare and that of her baby.

3.____

4. Ms. White is admitted to the hospital.
Because of the possibility of convulsive seizures, which of these articles should be readily available for Ms. White's care?

4.____

A. Oxygen and suction machine
B. Suction machine and mouth care tray
C. Mouth care tray and venous cutdown set
D. Venous cutdown set and oxygen

5. The next morning, Ms. White tells the nurse that she thinks she is beginning to have contractions.
For the timing of uterine contractions, it is recommended that she place

   A. her hands on the upper part of the abdomen, on opposite sides, and curve them somewhat around the uterine fundus
   B. the heel of the hand on the abdomen, just above the umbilicus, and press firmly
   C. her hand flat on the abdomen over the uterine fundus, with the fingers apart, and press lightly
   D. her hand in the middle of the upper part of the abdomen and then move the hand several times to different parts of the upper abdomen during each contraction

5.____

6. Ms. White goes into labor.
If Ms. White were to complain of a severe headache while she is in labor, the nurse should INITIALLY

   A. put Ms. White flat in bed with one pillow under her head
   B. take Ms. White's blood pressure
   C. check Ms. White's chart to determine whether she has recently received an analgesic
   D. count the fetal heart rate

6.____

7. Ms. White delivers a girl. Baby White's Apgar score at 1 minute is 8.
The CHIEF purpose of the first Apgar scoring of a newborn is to

   A. obtain a baseline for comparison with the infant's future development
   B. evaluate the efficiency of the infant's vital functions
   C. assess the effectiveness of the initial care given to the infant
   D. determine the presence of gross malformations in the infant

7.____

8. Ms. White is transferred to the postpartum unit, and Baby Girl White is transferred to the newborn nursery. Ms. White had a normal vaginal delivery, but is having difficulty voiding in the early postpartum.
The cause of her difficulty is MOST likely due to

   A. decreased abdominal pressure and trauma to the trigone of the bladder
   B. decreased blood volume and increased production of estrogen and progesterone
   C. increased bladder tone and emotional stress
   D. constriction of the kidney pelves and ureters

8.____

9. Ms. White is bottle-feeding her baby.
Which of these manifestations developing in her nipples or breasts on the third day after delivery would be NORMAL?

   A. Decrease in secretion from the breasts
   B. Engorgement of the breasts
   C. Inversion of the nipples
   D. Tenderness and redness of the nipples

9.____

Questions 10-11.

DIRECTIONS: Questions 10 and 11 are to be answered on the basis of the following information.

Ms. Ellen Stone, an 18-year-old primigravida, is brought to the hospital in early active labor. She has received no antepartal care during her pregnancy.

10. Which of these observations of Ms. Stone would be the MOST reliable indication that she is in true labor?

    A. Strong, intermittent uterine contractions
    B. Progressive cervical effacement and dilatation
    C. Rupture of the membranes
    D. Engagement of the presenting part

11. During the first stage of Ms. Stone's labor, which of these measures by the nurse would be MOST supportive of her?

    A. Administering sufficient analgesia to minimize pain from uterine contractions and encouraging her to remain on her back
    B. Keeping her informed about the progress of her labor and helping her to relax between contractions
    C. Having her hold on to the nurse's hand during the height of contractions and reminding her to breathe rapidly with her mouth open
    D. Telling her to bear down with her contractions and instructing her to sleep between contractions

Questions 12-21.

DIRECTIONS: Questions 12 through 21 are to be answered on the basis of the following information.

Ms. Karen Newman, a 26-year-old multipara, is pregnant. Her obstetric history includes 2 full-term pregnancies terminating in normal deliveries and, prior to her present pregnancy, a spontaneous abortion at 14 weeks' gestation. She is receiving antepartal care from a private physician.

12. On the basis of Ms. Newman's obstetric history, she is designated as a gravida _____, para _____.

    A. III; II   B. III; IV   C. IV; II   D. IV; III

13. Ms. Newman weighs 152 lb. (68.95 kg.) at the end of the fourth month of gestation. Her weight before she became pregnant was 135 lb. (61.23 kg.), which was normal for her age and body build.
    It is justifiable to say that Ms. Newman's 17-lb. (7.72 kg.) weight gain for her stage of pregnancy is

    A. below average   B. average
    C. somewhat above average   D. excessive

14. Ms. Newman tells the nurse that her 2 1/2-year-old son, Danny, tends to be jealous and that she is worried about how he may react to the new baby.
    The nurse's reply should indicate that jealousy in a 2 1/2-year-old

    A. can be lessened by providing a mother-substitute for the child when the mother first returns home from the hospital
    B. can be suppressed if the child's contact with the new baby is restricted
    C. cannot be handled by reasoning with the child
    D. cannot be dealt with therapeutically

15. Ms. Newman is 2 weeks past term. She is admitted to the hospital for induction of labor with an oxytocic drug. Upon admission, Ms. Newman is permitted to have liquids by mouth.
    Which of these foods would probably be CONTRAINDICATED for her?

    A. Tea with lemon
    B. Ginger ale
    C. Milk
    D. Gelatin dessert

16. Which of these findings, if present in Ms. Newman, would it be ESSENTIAL for the registered nurse to report to the physician before the oxytocic infusion is started?

    A. Low backache
    B. A rise in blood pressure from 122/80 to 130/84
    C. An increase in pulse rate from 88 to 98
    D. Regular contractions of 60 seconds' duration

17. Ms. Newman has an intravenous infusion running, to which oxytocin injection (Pitocin) has been added.
    Which of these conditions would warrant IMMEDIATE discontinuation of Ms. Newman's intravenous infusion of Pitocin?

    A. Increase in show
    B. Rupture of the membranes
    C. A sustained uterine contraction
    D. A fetal heart rate of 120 during a contraction

18. Ms. Newman has an order for 100 mg. of meperidine (Demerol) hydrochloride.
    Which of these groups of signs in Ms. Newman would MOST clearly indicate that a dose of Demerol could be given to her with safety?
    Cervical dilatation, _____ cm.; presenting part at _____ station; uterine contractions q._____ minutes, lasting _____ seconds; fetal heart rate, _____ beats per minute.

    A. 3; 0; 10; 45; 100
    B. 4; 0; 3; 50; 172
    C. 5; -1; 5; 40; 144
    D. 7; -1; 2; 60; 120

19. In view of the fact that Ms. Newman had general anesthesia, it would be safe to start giving her oral fluids

    A. after she voids for the first time
    B. after she has coughed voluntarily
    C. when her pulse rate is 70 beats per minute
    D. when she has rested for about an hour after admission to the postpartum unit

20. Penicillin ointment rather than silver nitrate is used in the prophylactic eye care of Baby Boy Newman to

    A. promote a more lasting bacteriostatic effect
    B. gain a more rapid systemic effect
    C. administer therapeutic amounts with greater ease
    D. cause less irritation of the conjunctivae

21. Six weeks after the birth of her baby, Ms. Newman returns to the clinic for a routine follow-up visit. At the clinic, Ms. Newman says to the nurse, *Having so many children makes it very hard for us to manage, but my husband won't do anything to prevent me from getting pregnant. He gets angry when I even mention the idea.* Which of these approaches by the nurse is LIKELY to be MOST useful?

    A. Give Ms. Newman a pamphlet for her husband that describes various contraceptive methods.
    B. Ask Ms. Newman to have her husband accompany her to the clinic to talk with the nurse about contraception.
    C. Refer Ms. Newman to an agency that provides family planning services.
    D. Find out from Ms. Newman if her husband would be willing to accept a method of contraception that would not involve him directly.

Questions 22-30.

DIRECTIONS: Questions 22 through 30 are to be answered on the basis of the following information.

Ms. Barbara Wing, 21 years old, attends the antepartal clinic for the first time when she has missed two menstrual periods. The physician determines that she is pregnant and finds her to be in good health. This is her first pregnancy.

22. During Ms. Wing's initial conference with the registered nurse, she mentions that although she usually feels well, there are times when she feels tired.
Which of these responses by the nurse would be BEST?

    A. Fatigue is normal when the body is adjusting to the pregnant state. Let's talk about your daily schedule so we can plan extra rest for you.
    B. It will be necessary for you to cut down on your usual activities and try to get more rest. About how many hours of sleep do you get at night?
    C. Your fatigue is probably due to hormonal changes that occur in early pregnancy. As your body adapts to the demands of your developing baby, this feeling will pass.
    D. Your fatigue at this time indicates that you probably will have to give special consideration to rest, and possibly even to diet, throughout your pregnancy.

23. Ms. Wing is to include extra amounts of vitamin C in her diet.
She should be instructed that the juice that has the
LEAST vitamin C per average serving is

    A. canned apple   B. canned tomato
    C. fresh grapefruit   D. frozen orange

24. Ms. Wing's pregnancy progresses normally.
    In the latter part of the third trimester, Ms. Wing should be advised to take which of these precautions relative to bathing?

    A. Take sponge baths exclusively
    B. Avoid using bath salts
    C. Bathe only in tepid water
    D. Place nonskid material at the bottom of the bathtub

25. Ms. Wing is at term and in early active labor when she is brought to the hospital by her husband. Mr. and Ms. Wing attended a series of preparation for childbirth classes. Such a program is MOST likely to be successful if the

    A. parents and the medical and nursing staff have accepted the philosophy, principles, and techniques of the classes
    B. physician is present during labor and gives support to the mother
    C. nurse who is to stay with the mother during labor and delivery is prepared to assist the father in coaching his wife
    D. mother and father are truly prepared for their roles during labor and delivery

26. The nurse makes all of the following observations of Ms. Wing during the second stage of her labor.
    Which one would be of GREATEST significance in terms of her welfare and that of her baby?
    A(n)

    A. sudden increase in blood-tinged show
    B. change in the baseline blood pressure from 110/80 to 90/60
    C. fetal heart rate of 152 to 160 beats per minute between contractions
    D. increase in maternal pulse rate from 90 to 95 beats per minute during contractions

27. Ms. Wing has an episiotomy and delivers a girl weighing 7 lb. 5 oz. (3,317 gm.).
    Which of these observations of Ms. Wing would indicate that normal placental separation is occurring? She has

    A. hardening and thickening of the exposed portion of the umbilical cord, softening of the uterine fundus, and a steady stream of blood from the vagina
    B. strong uterine contractions, recession of the uterine fundus below the symphysis pubis, and temporary absence of vaginal bleeding
    C. gaping of the vulva in conjunction with strong uterine contractions, rapid enlargement of the uterus, and oozing of blood from the vagina
    D. increased protrusion of the umbilical cord from the vagina, the uterus' becoming globular-shaped, and a sudden spurting of blood from the vagina

28. Ms. Wing is transferred to the postpartum unit, and Baby Girl Wing is transferred to the newborn nursery.
    In examining Ms. Wing's episiotomy incision, which of these positions would be appropriate for the patient and would BEST help to minimize strain on the sutures?

    A. Prone
    B. Knee-chest
    C. Sim's
    D. Trendelenburg

29. Which of these measures, if carried out before Baby Girl Wing's discharge, will PROBABLY contribute to Ms. Wing's confidence in her ability to care for her baby?

   A. Having Ms. Wing observe demonstrations of infant care in which equipment commonly found in the home is used
   B. Having Ms. Wing take care of the baby in the hospital under the guidance of the registered nurse
   C. Arranging for Mr. Wing to learn how to assist Ms. Wing with caring for the baby
   D. Arranging to have the community health nurse visit with Ms. Wing and discuss areas that are of concern to Ms. Wing

30. Mr. and Ms. Wing discuss birth control with the nurse. In selecting a method of birth control, the Wings should give priority to

   A. Ms. Wing's age
   B. the length of their marriage
   C. the technique they find most acceptable
   D. the success rate of a particular method

KEY (CORRECT ANSWERS)

1.	D	16.	D
2.	D	17.	C
3.	B	18.	C
4.	A	19.	B
5.	C	20.	D
6.	B	21.	D
7.	B	22.	A
8.	A	23.	A
9.	B	24.	D
10.	B	25.	A
11.	B	26.	B
12.	C	27.	D
13.	D	28.	C
14.	C	29.	B
15.	C	30.	C

EXAMINATION SECTION
TEST 1

DIRECTIONS: Each question or incomplete statement is followed by several suggested answers or completions. Select the one that BEST answers the question or completes the statement. *PRINT THE LETTER OF THE CORRECT ANSWER IN THE SPACE AT THE RIGHT.*

Questions 1-2.

DIRECTIONS: Questions 1 and 2 are to be answered on the basis of the following information.

Mrs. Jones, who has been diagnosed with severe preeclampsia, is placed on bedrest. An IV of lactated Ringer's solution has been started.

1. The nurse inserted an in-dwelling catheter to measure urine output

    A. because some urine may be lost when voided on a bed pan
    B. because urine output should be measured hourly to detect increasing oliguria
    C. to measure 24-hour urine for proteins
    D. to keep bed from getting wet

2. What position should the nurse encourage Mrs. Jones to maintain as she is at high risk with severe preeclampsia?

    A. Left lateral recumbent
    B. Semi-Fowler's
    C. Supine
    D. Right lateral

3. Mrs. Arnold is 34 years old. She is admitted to the hospital for a subtotal hysterectomy. She has a history of fibroid tumors.
   The MOST common symptom of fibroid tumors is

    A. menorrhagia
    B. bleeding in-between periods
    C. premenstrual pain
    D. premenstrual edema

4. A patient admitted for a total hysterectomy asks the nurse caring for her if her ovaries will be removed during the operation.
   The nurse's BEST response is:

    A. The ovaries remain intact, but the cervix and uterus will be removed
    B. It is better to remove the ovaries as they serve no purpose
    C. Ask your doctor; I am not the doctor
    D. It doesn't really matter whether they leave them or remove them

5. Post-operatively, a patient of total hysterectomy should be told that

    A. she should abstain from sexual intercourse for the rest of her life
    B. dancing and heavy exercises should be avoided because of pelvic congestion
    C. weight gain frequently occurs
    D. atrophy of breasts is common

6. A patient asks the nurse what pap smears signify. The nurse's reply should be that

   A. it signifies cancer, if positive
   B. abnormal cells seen in a pap smear may be caused by conditions other than cancer
   C. it is always done on patients with cervical cancer
   D. all of the above

7. Mrs. Stanford, a 68-year-old woman, had a hysterectomy performed vaginally. The nursing care in the first 24 hours postoperatively should include

   A. oral administration of fluids
   B. frequent observation of dressing
   C. placing her in semi-Fowler's position
   D. frequent changing of perineal pads

8. Which of the following is TRUE regarding a pap smear preparation?

   A. A douche should be done on the morning of the exam.
   B. It should be taken during menstruation.
   C. Specimen should be allowed to dry before fixing solution is applied to slide.
   D. Tub baths are suggested for 5 days before the exam.

9. The cure rate for cervical cancer is a

   A. five-year survival rate of 75% if treated in early stages
   B. 100% cure rate if treated surgically when detected in early stages
   C. five-year survival rate of only 50%
   D. none of the above

10. A 60-year-old woman with a malignant tumor of the breast is admitted for modified radical mastectomy.
    To provide support, the nurse should

    A. plan experiences for her that are constructive
    B. help identify her problems and solutions
    C. give information as to how to handle her problem
    D. tell her of her strength and progress

11. A patient tells the nurse that she was treated for syphilis at her first antepartum visit, when it was discovered. The patient worries that, even though she has been told that she is now cured, her baby will be affected.
    How should the nurse reply?

    A. No matter what, the baby will be affected.
    B. The baby will not be affected because you can have syphilis only once.
    C. The baby will probably not be affected, especially if you don't get syphilis again while you are pregnant.
    D. Do not worry about the baby at this time.

12. When the diagnosis of uterine atony is made for persistent uterine bleeding, it can be managed by massaging the uterus to stimulate contractions and administering   12.____

    A. magnesium sulphate
    B. oxytocic medications
    C. vitamin K to the mother
    D. dextrose ultravenously

13. A woman who is pregnant for the first time wants to know about afterpains. You should tell her that afterpains are MORE common in   13.____

    A. primiparas who are not breastfeeding
    B. mothers who are pumping their breasts
    C. multipara mothers who are nursing
    D. multiparas who are not nursing

14. A woman who was using an oral contraceptive stopped taking it six months ago, and now her menses are two weeks late.
    The MOST probable sign of pregnancy would be   14.____

    A. amenorrhea
    B. frequent urination
    C. tender breasts
    D. positive pregnancy test

15. Which of the following is TRUE about pregnancy tests done on urine?   15.____

    A. Presence of estrogen in urine confirms pregnancy.
    B. Presence of alpha human chorionic gonadotropin confirms pregnancy.
    C. Presence of beta human chorionic gonadotropins confirms pregnancy until proven otherwise.
    D. Home tests are less reliable because of errors in use.

16. A pregnant woman who had syphilis was treated at 10 weeks of pregnancy with penicillin.
    The newborn baby would be MOST likely to   16.____

    A. have syphilis
    B. have positive titre at birth
    C. be premature
    D. be an asymptomatic carrier

17. The result of the growing uterus on the bladder is   17.____

    A. frequency
    B. urgency
    C. dysurea
    D. flank pain

18. A woman in her first trimester was admitted to the hospital for abdominal pain. She was told that she has 1+ sugar in her urine. She asks you, *Am I diabetic?*
    Your BEST response would be to   18.____

    A. tell her that she might be diabetic
    B. reassure the mother that this is a normal finding during the first trimester
    C. tell the mother that you need some more testing
    D. notify an endocrinologist and let him/her talk to the woman

19. The PROBABLE day of ovulation for a woman with a 30-day regular menstrual cycle is the _____ th day of the cycle.   19.____

    A. 6
    B. 14
    C. 16
    D. 10

20. A 12 weeks pregnant woman comes to the emergency room with vaginal bleeding. You are there with the physician, and you notice on examination that the cervix is 2 cm dilated.
    The MOST likely diagnosis is _____ abortion.

    A. inevitable
    B. missed
    C. threatened
    D. incomplete

Questions 21-22.

DIRECTIONS: Questions 21 and 22 are to be answered on the basis of the following information.

Mrs. Smith is 35 weeks pregnant and complaining of hemorrhoidal pain.

21. Pregnant women are prone to hemorrhoids because

    A. the gravid uterus exerts pressure on the large intestine
    B. vascularity throughout the pelvic region is increased
    C. of constipation
    D. all of the above

22. Mrs. Smith also wants something to relieve her anal discomfort immediately. What would you suggest?

    A. Wait for the physician to come
    B. Reassure the client that this is normal in pregnancy
    C. Use of an ice bag or cold witch hazel compress
    D. Avoid knee-chest position

23. While assessing a client for third trimester bleeding due to abruptio placentae, _____ is contraindicated.

    A. monitoring of vital signs
    B. bedside assurance to client
    C. abdominal exam for signs of rigidity and tenderness
    D. vaginal exam to evaluate the labor

24. Complications developing from abruptio placentae include

    A. temperature of 100° F
    B. disseminated intravascular coagulopathy
    C. decreased urine output
    D. seizure activity

Questions 25-26.

DIRECTIONS: Questions 25 and 26 are to be answered on the basis of the following information.

A pregnant woman, gravida 4 para 3, is admitted to labor and delivery with bright red vaginal bleeding. She has a history of short labor and elevated blood pressure since 28 weeks of gestation. She is 36 weeks pregnant now, amniotic fluid is leaking, and blood pressure is 150/100.

25. The MOST likely diagnosis is

    A. chronic hypertension
    B. pregnancy-induced hypertension
    C. abruptio placentae
    D. multiple pregnancy

26. The MOST likely cause of this patient's condition is

    A. chronic hypertension
    B. pregnancy-induced hypertension
    C. threatened abortion
    D. multiple pregnancy

27. A woman is admitted to labor and delivery. In active labor, meconium-stained amniotic fluid is leaking.
    You should IMMEDIATELY

    A. contact a physician
    B. apply fetal heart tone monitor and assess fetal well-being
    C. start amnio infusion
    D. prepare for an emergency cesarean section

28. A primipara is admitted to the hospital because of pregnancy-induced hypertension at 28 weeks gestation. She is 37 years old. Amniocentesis is normal.
    The MOST appropriate nursing action at this time would be to

    A. record vital signs
    B. start an intravenous line
    C. administer antihypertensive drugs
    D. call the physician immediately

29. A primipara at 38 weeks of gestation calls the labor and delivery room at midnight to say that she is in labor. You happen to be attending the phone.
    Which of the following signs will tell you that she is TRULY in labor?

    A. She has nausea and vomiting.
    B. She has contractions which are faint and not increasing in duration and frequency.
    C. Her contractions are increasing in duration and frequency.
    D. She can walk easily with the contractions.

30. A woman who has been pushing for the last 12 hours is exhausted, but now, in the transition phase, she shouts at her husband and asks him to leave her alone.
    The BEST nursing action at this time would be to

    A. tell the father to leave the room
    B. accept this behavior as normal in this situation
    C. tell the client to keep quiet
    D. tell the father to leave the room now and come back later

KEY (CORRECT ANSWERS)

1.	B	16.	B
2.	A	17.	A
3.	A	18.	B
4.	A	19.	C
5.	B	20.	A
6.	B	21.	D
7.	D	22.	C
8.	C	23.	D
9.	B	24.	B
10.	B	25.	C
11.	C	26.	B
12.	B	27.	B
13.	C	28.	A
14.	D	29.	C
15.	C	30.	B

TEST 2

DIRECTIONS: Each question or incomplete statement is followed by several suggested answers or completions. Select the one that BEST answers the question or completes the statement. *PRINT THE LETTER OF THE CORRECT ANSWER IN THE SPACE AT THE RIGHT.*

1. The nurse asks a postpartum mother about uterine discharge on the second day. The EXPECTED answer would be lochia _____, i.e., _____ discharge.

    A. serosa; pinkish
    B. rubra; dark red
    C. alba; creamy
    D. verde; green

2. All of the following are postpartal changes in the uterus EXCEPT

    A. involution of the uterus
    B. immediately after delivery, top of fundus is several finger breadths above the umbilicus
    C. twelve hours after delivery, fundus of the uterus is one finger breadth above the umbilicus
    D. fundus descends into the pelvis approximately two finger breadths per day

3. After having a baby, a mother who is not breastfeeding will PROBABLY resume menstruation in _____ weeks.

    A. 12   B. 8   C. 6   D. 4

4. All of the following are changes that occur in the gastrointestinal system after delivery EXCEPT

    A. immediately after delivery, hunger is common
    B. gastrointestinal tract is sluggish and hypoactive
    C. heartburn is common
    D. constipation may be a problem

5. A postpartum mother is complaining of urinary retention. You explain to the mother that this is normal.
   Other changes that occur in the urinary system postpartum include

    A. increased bladder capacity and decreased sensitivity to pressure leading to urinary retention
    B. hematuria after delivery
    C. bladder is edematous and hyperemic
    D. all of the above

6. All of the following are postpartal high risk factors EXCEPT

    A. preeclampsia/eclampsia
    B. cesarean birth
    C. abruptio placenta
    D. twin pregnancy

7. A 28-year-old gravida 1 para 0 mother has delivered a baby weighing 10 lbs. via vaginal delivery, which was uneventful. Two hours later, the nurse notices continuous bleeding. This condition could be caused by

    A. uterine atony
    B. lacerations
    C. retained placental tissue
    D. all of the above

8. Predisposing factors for puerperal infections do NOT include

   A. twin pregnancy
   B. premature rupture of membranes
   C. prolonged labor
   D. antepartal infection

9. Local infections acquired during pregnancy or delivery may extend via the lymphatics into the pelvic organs and may cause all of the following EXCEPT

   A. salpingitis/oophoritis
   B. thrombophlebitis
   C. septicemia
   D. pneumonia

10. The BEST nursing intervention to prevent puerperal infections is to

    A. maintain meticulous aseptic techniques during labor and delivery
    B. assess and treat antepartal infections
    C. avoid prolonged labor
    D. all of the above

11. Mastitis, or invasion of the breast tissue by pathogenic organisms, is a common complaint after delivery.
    The MOST common organism causing mastitis is

    A. group B streptococcus
    B. staphylococcus aureus
    C. meisseria gonorrhea
    D. escherechia coli

12. To PREVENT complications of mastitis, the nurse should

    A. teach the mother how to cleanse the breasts and nipple
    B. provide instructions regarding MASSE cream
    C. explain the importance of wearing a supporting bra
    D. all of the above

13. Which of the following statements is CORRECT regarding postpartum psychosis?

    A. Depression is the most common type of psychiatric disorder seen after birth.
    B. Pregnancy is usually not a precipitating factor/event that leads to the crisis.
    C. Most mothers who suffer from postpartum psychosis do not have a previous history of psychiatric illness.
    D. Psychotic complication is common.

14. A woman who has undergone cesarean section is complaining of headaches, which is not unusual.
    What would you suggest for this patient at this time?

    A. Maintain bedrest in left lateral position
    B. Bedrest in a flat or recumbent position
    C. Sit in the bed for 15 minutes every 3 hours
    D. Try to ambulate as soon as possible

15. A mother just delivered a baby. While doing episiotomy repair, the physician noticed hemorrhage. He immediately ordered a transfusion.
    While waiting for the blood, the BEST factor to check to evaluate the patient's status is

    A. blood pressure
    B. amount of bleeding
    C. repeated hematocrit level
    D. level of alertness

    15._____

16. A 22-year-old woman just delivered her baby vaginally. She had an episiotomy. When she was moved to the recovery room, she started shaking.
    An APPROPRIATE nursing action at this time would be to

    A. notify the delivering physician immediately
    B. give interavenous fluids
    C. administer oxygen
    D. cover the women with warm blankets

    16._____

17. A mother who delivered a baby this morning and had an episiotomy is complaining of pain at the episiotomy site. On inspection, you notice that the episiotomy site is edematous, sutures are intact, and no hematomas are noted.
    What would you suggest the mother do?

    A. Apply ice packs to the perineum area
    B. Take sitz baths as desired
    C. Take demerol to relieve pain
    D. Postpartal Kegel exercises

    17._____

18. The ONLY safe, non-prescription contraceptive method while a woman is lactating and before normal uterine involution is

    A. condoms and contraceptive foam
    B. intrauterine device
    C. diaphragm and jelly
    D. oral contraceptives.

    18._____

19. A postpartum 28-year-old woman develops a fever of 100° F, is urinating a lot, and is diaphoretic.
    The BEST nursing intervention at this time would be to

    A. notify the physician immediately
    B. reassure the mother that these are normal findings in the first 24 hours after delivery
    C. send blood for cultures and complete blood count
    D. stop the mother from breastfeeding because she might be infected

    19._____

20. A 27-year-old diabetic mother just delivered a baby. The nurse knows that she is at high risk for postpartum bleeding.
    The MOST frequent cause of uterine postpartal hemorrhage is

    A. uterine inertia
    C. lacerations
    B. uterine atony
    D. retained placental tissue

    20._____

21. All of the following are correct regarding mothers with postpartal hemorrhage who are breastfeeding EXCEPT

    A. iron supplement should be given
    B. breastfeeding is contraindicated in postpartal hemorrhage
    C. the maternal diet should be high in protein and iron-rich foods
    D. fatigue is common

22. An RH negative primipara mother just delivered an RH positive baby. Which of the following tests would show that she is NOT sensitized?

    A. Negative Klie Hower Bethke test
    B. Positive Coombs test on maternal blood
    C. Negative Coombs test on maternal blood
    D. Maternal hemoglobin and hematocrit

23. An RH negative mother with an RH positive fetus is to receive RhoGAM, which

    A. attaches to maternal red blood cells and destroys them
    B. attaches to antibodies produced by the mother against RH positive fetal red blood cells
    C. attaches to RH positive fetal red blood cells in maternal circulation and destroys them before sensitization occurs
    D. destroys both maternal and fetal red blood cells

Questions 24-25.

DIRECTIONS: Questions 24 and 25 are to be answered on the basis of the following information.

Mrs. Stein just delivered a baby. She was told to do Kegel's exercises.

24. Kegel's exercises are good for

    A. relieving episiotomy pain
    B. controlling urethral sphincter
    C. enhancing coital pleasure
    D. all of the above

25. Mrs. Stein also asks if you can suggest any other exercises which would help relieve her menstrual cramps.
    What would you suggest?

    A. Kegel's exercises
    B. Pelvic rock exercises
    C. Take aspirin and no exercise
    D. Tell her to contact her gynecologist

26. A mother who delivered a baby this morning tells you that she and her husband want to have tubal ligation done.
Tubal ligation

    A. can easily be reversed anytime
    B. is an in-patient procedure
    C. is not as safe as vasectomy
    D. removes the worry about pregnancy

27. Mutual regulation is a phase of mother-infant interaction which occurs

    A. during touching activities, in face position
    B. when there is bonding between parent and infant
    C. during the phase of feeding, bathing, and comforting the new baby
    D. when mother first touches the baby

28. All of the following factors influence maternal-infant attachment EXCEPT

    A. relationship with own parents
    B. previous experience with infants
    C. social, economic, and developmental level of mother
    D. none of the above

29. As an essential part of the attachment process, the mother begins to *discover* her infant. This includes identification of _____ of the baby.

    A. congenital defects
    B. physical characteristics and bodily processes
    C. sickness
    D. rash on the face

30. Regarding parent reaction to the birth of a premature infant, the first period is the period of disorganization, which is characterized by

    A. guilt, anger, and sorrow
    B. beginning of problem solving
    C. need of more information to solve the crisis
    D. decreases anxiety

KEY (CORRECT ANSWERS)

1. B
2. A
3. A
4. A
5. B

6. B
7. D
8. C
9. B
10. B

11. C
12. B
13. C
14. D
15. C

16. B
17. A
18. B
19. C
20. A

21. D
22. C
23. D
24. B
25. C

26. B
27. B
28. A
29. C
30. B

EXAMINATION SECTION
TEST 1

DIRECTIONS: Each question or incomplete statement is followed by several suggested answers or completions. Select the one that BEST answers the question or completes the statement. *PRINT THE LETTER OF THE CORRECT ANSWER IN THE SPACE AT THE RIGHT.*

1. Mothers of infants and toddlers should be instructed that diets for their children that include milk at the expense of other foods are MOST likely to result in the development of a deficiency in

    A. iron
    B. carbohydrate
    C. vitamin D
    D. vitamin K

    1.____

2. A 1-week-old boy, weighing 6 pounds, has just been returned to the pediatric unit after having surgery for an intestinal obstruction. He has nasogastric suction and is receiving intravenous fluids via a venous cutdown. In addition to meeting the infant's special needs, which of these measures would be ESSENTIAL?

    A. Restraining all four of the baby's extremities
    B. Handling the baby as little as possible
    C. Explaining the equipment used in the baby's treatment to his mother so that she can assist the nurse with his care
    D. Spending time stroking the baby

    2.____

3. A mother makes all of these comments about her infant daughter to the physician. Which one describes a characteristic MORE likely to be observed in an infant with hypothyroidism than in a normal 3-month-old infant?

    A. She smiles a lot.
    B. She's so good and she never cries.
    C. She notices her toys and she knows my voice.
    D. She seems to spend a great deal of time watching her hands.

    3.____

Questions 4-7.

DIRECTIONS: Questions 4 through 7 are to be answered on the basis of the following information.

Bruce Alfonse, 9 years old, has an acute asthmatic attack and is admitted to the hospital because he did not respond to treatment in the emergency room. He has had bronchial asthma since early childhood.

4. Bruce is to receive 100 mg. of aminophylline intravenously.
   If the ampules of aminophylline available on Bruce's unit contain aminophylline gr. 7 1/2 in 10 cc. of solution, how much solution from the ampule will contain 100 mg. of aminophylline?

    A. 2 cc.   B. 4 cc.   C. 6 cc.   D. 8 cc.

    4.____

5. Which of these events in Bruce's life would be MOST likely to cause an increase in the frequency and intensity of his asthmatic attacks?

    5.____

133

A. Ms. Alfonse's buying new furniture for Bruce's bedroom
B. The Alfonse's moving to another city
C. Mr. Alfonse's being away from home on business for several days
D. Bruce's favorite grandparent's coming to visit for a week

6. An IMPORTANT objective of the medical and nursing management of Bruce should be to help him to

   A. accept the fact that he cannot be like other children and that he will have to limit his goals
   B. accept his condition and live a productive life
   C. understand the underlying cause of his condition
   D. accept being dependent upon his mother until he is in his middle teens

7. The nurse is planning Bruce's care.
Consideration should be given to the fact that most normal 8-year-olds

   A. prefer to associate with a peer of the same sex
   B. seek opportunities for socializing with older boys
   C. enjoy small heterosexual groups
   D. function best as a member of a large group of somewhat younger boys and girls

Questions 8-13.

DIRECTIONS: Questions 8 through 13 are to be answered on the basis of the following information.

Jeff Green, age 2 1/2, sustained a simple fracture of the shaft of the left femur when he fell down stairs at home. Upon his admission to the hospital, Jeff is placed in Bryant's traction.

8. Among the equipment used in the application of Bryant's traction is

   A. adhesive material on the skin of both limbs
   B. metal calipers in the malleoli of both ankles
   C. a Kirschner wire in the affected femur
   D. a Thomas splint on the fractured extremity

9. During his first two days in the hospital, Jeff lies quietly, sucks his thumb, and does not cry.
It is MOST justifiable to say that he

   A. has made a good adjustment to the traction
   B. is accustomed to being disciplined at home
   C. has confidence in the nurses caring for him
   D. is experiencing anxiety

10. Prior to his admission, Jeff was partially bowel-trained, but now he defecates involuntarily.
The nurse's approach to this problem should be based on which of these assessments?

    A. What is Jeff's reaction to his soiling
    B. How compulsive is Jeff about cleanliness

C. Is Jeff too young for bowel training
D. Is bowel training important for Jeff

11. Ms. Green is upset because when she comes to visit, Jeff turns his head away from her and holds his arms out to the nurse.
It is probably MOST justifiable to say that Jeff

   A. is angry with his mother for leaving him in the hospital
   B. is testing the relationship between his mother and the nurse
   C. now has a stronger emotional tie with the nurse than with his mother
   D. is consciously trying to make his mother jealous

11._____

12. One day when the nurse offers Jeff a cookie, he says *No!* and at the same time holds out his hand for it.
Which of these interpretations of Jeff's behavior is PROBABLY justifiable?

   A. His mother has forbidden sweets, and he is in conflict about accepting any.
   B. He is confused about the meaning of yes and no.
   C. His negativism is a beginning attempt at independence.
   D. He is unaccustomed to being offered choices.

12._____

13. To prevent accidents such as Jeff's among toddlers, which one of the following measures would probably help MOST?

   A. Having carpeting on stairs
   B. Using adjustable gates on stairways
   C. Providing the toddler with a plentiful supply of play materials in one room
   D. Keeping the toddler in a playpen placed near the mother's work area

13._____

Questions 14-19.

DIRECTIONS: Questions 14 through 18 are to be answered on the basis of the following information.

Adam Crane, 13 years old, is admitted to the hospital for treatment of acute rheumatic fever. He is placed on bed rest.

14. Adam MOST probably has which of these groups of symptoms that are characteristic of acute rheumatic fever?

   A. Swelling of the fingers, petechiae, and general malaise
   B. Nodules overlying bony prominences, dependent edema, and elevated blood pressure
   C. Bleeding gums, dyspnea, and failure to gain weight
   D. Fever, rash, and migratory joint pain

14._____

15. Adam is receiving a corticosteroid drug.
He should be observed for common side effects of this type of drug therapy, such as

   A. hypotension   B. weight loss
   C. pallor   D. acne

15._____

16. An oral potassium preparation is ordered for Adam. The CHIEF purpose of this drug for him is to

16._____

A. promote excretion of bacterial toxins
B. prevent hypokalemia
C. enhance the action of the corticosteroid drug
D. reduce the electrical potential of the cardiac conduction system

17. Adam's blood tests include all of the following results. Which of these results would be MOST indicative of improvement in his condition?

    A. Positive C-reactive protein
    B. Hemoglobin, 14.0 Gm. per 100 cc. of blood
    C. White blood cell count, 11,000 per cu. mm. of blood
    D. Decreasing erythrocyte sedimentation rate

18. Permanent functional impairment would MOST likely result if Adam developed

    A. erythema marginatum   B. polyarthritis
    C. carditis   D. subcutaneous nodules

19. Recurrent attacks of rheumatic fever in Adam can BEST be prevented by

    A. keeping him on prophylactic drug therapy for an indefinite period
    B. including foods in his diet that are rich in vitamins and minerals
    C. improving his family's socioeconomic condition
    D. providing daily afternoon rest periods for him for about a year after recovery from an acute attack

Questions 20-25.

DIRECTIONS: Questions 20 through 25 are to be answered on the basis of the following information.

Daniel Rich, 6 weeks old, is admitted to the pediatric unit with pyloric stenosis. He is to have a pyloromyotomy.

20. Daniel's parents tell the nurse that they do not quite understand what the doctor has told them about the operation, and they ask for clarification.
    Which of these explanations to the parents would be MOST appropriate?

    A. Daniel's stomach is contracted and its capacity diminished, making it necessary for the doctor to dilate it with instruments.
    B. Nerves have produced contraction of certain muscles in Daniel's stomach called sphincters, and these nerves must be cut in order to produce relaxation.
    C. Constricting bands of tissue in the middle of Daniel's stomach, which are causing vomiting, will be resected.
    D. The doctor will make a cut in a tight muscle at the bottom of Daniel's stomach, which has caused his symptoms.

21. Preoperatively, Daniel is to receive 0.15 mg. (gr. 1/400) of atropine sulfate.
    If a vial containing 0.4 mg. (gr. 1/150) in 1 cc. of solution is used to prepare Daniel's dose, how much of the stock solution should be given to him?
    _____ cc.

    A. 0.28   B. 0.33   C. 0.38   D. 0.43

22. Daniel should be observed for early symptoms of side effects of atropine, which include   22.____

    A. vomiting and subnormal temperature
    B. lethargy and bradycardia
    C. rapid respirations and flushed skin
    D. muscle spasms and diaphoresis

23. Daniel has a pyloromyotomy.   23.____
    Assuming that Daniel's operation is successful, his parents should be informed that his convalescence can be expected to be

    A. *gradual,* with the persistence of mild preoperative symptoms for a few weeks
    B. *prolonged,* with gradual reduction and eventual disappearance of preoperative symptoms over a period of a few months
    C. *brief,* but with periodic recurrence of preoperative symptoms during his first 6 months of life
    D. *rapid,* and characterized by the absence of preoperative symptoms

24. Daniel is now 8 weeks old. He should be expected to   24.____

    A. cry when a stranger approaches
    B. pay attention to a voice
    C. laugh aloud
    D. make sounds such as *ba-ba* and *da-da*

25. In response to Ms. Rich's questions, the nurse discusses with her the introduction of new foods into Daniel's diet.   25.____
    Which of these suggestions by the nurse would be MOST appropriate?

    A. Whenever a new food is added to Daniel's diet, decrease the amount of milk offered to him.
    B. Give Daniel new foods one at a time.
    C. Allow Daniel to touch each new solid food before he tastes it.
    D. Mix new foods with a small amount of some food Daniel has previously had.

KEY (CORRECT ANSWERS)

1.	A	11.	A
2.	D	12.	C
3.	B	13.	B
4.	A	14.	D
5.	B	15.	D
6.	B	16.	B
7.	A	17.	D
8.	A	18.	C
9.	D	19.	A
10.	A	20.	D

21. C
22. C
23. D
24. B
25. B

TEST 2

DIRECTIONS: Each question or incomplete statement is followed by several suggested answers or completions. Select the one that BEST answers the question or completes the statement. *PRINT THE LETTER OF THE CORRECT ANSWER IN THE SPACE AT THE RIGHT.*

1. Parents are given information relative to the nutrition of normal newborn infants. Which of the following statements is INACCURATE? 1.____

    A. Formulas made of modified cow's milk are well absorbed.
    B. A high protein intake assures a rapid growth rate.
    C. The total daily intake of nutrients is more important than the size or frequency of individual feedings.
    D. Infants born of well-nourished mothers are likely to have adequate stores of nutrients at birth.

2. A 3-year-old has nephrosis and marked ascites. In which position is she likely to be MOST comfortable? 2.____

    A. Semi-Fowler's   B. Sims'
    C. Dorsal recumbent   D. Prone

3. A 5-year-old with leukemia is to be discharged because his condition is in a state of remission. 3.____
   It will be MOST helpful to the child when he is at home if his parents understand that

    A. the child's condition is terminal, and it will be their responsibility to make him as happy as possible without making demands upon him
    B. they should guide their child, encouraging him and setting limits for him, so that he may develop to his full potential
    C. it will not be necessary for them to control their child's behavior because his condition makes him aware of his own limitations
    D. it will be important for them to develop a carefully planned schedule for the child that will conserve his strength

Questions 4-7.

DIRECTIONS: Questions 4 through 7 are to be answered on the basis of the following information.

   Josh Greene, 9 1/2 months old, is admitted to the hospital. He has a provisional diagnosis of intussusception.

4. Josh MOST probably has which of these symptoms that are characteristic manifestations of the onset of intussusception in an infant? 4.____

    A. Abdominal distention and coffee-ground vomitus
    B. Hyperpyrexia and rectal prolapse
    C. Passage of large amount of flatus associated with straining
    D. Paroxysmal abdominal pain accompanied by screaming

5. When the physician tells Mr. and Ms. Greene that immediate surgery will be necessary if Josh's diagnosis is confirmed, they are reluctant to give permission for the operation.
   If surgery is not performed soon after a diagnosis of intussusception is made, which of these conditions is LIKELY to result?

   A. Chronic ulcerative colitis
   B. Megacolon
   C. Meckel's diverticulum
   D. Gangrene of the bowel

6. A barium enema is ordered to help confirm Josh's diagnosis. An additional reason why a barium enema is ordered for Josh at this time is that it may result in

   A. elimination of offending toxins
   B. diminution of microbial flora of the intestine in preparation for surgery
   C. control of bleeding due to the barium's astringent effect on the bowel lining
   D. reduction of the telescoped bowel segment

7. Josh has intussusception, and the condition is corrected by surgery. His recovery is satisfactory.
   When Josh begins to feel better, the play material that would probably be MOST appropriate for him is a

   A. mobile
   B. beanbag
   C. roly-poly animal with a weighted base
   D. tinker toy with parts securely fastened

Questions 8-15.

DIRECTIONS: Questions 8 through 15 are to be answered on the basis of the following information.

Amy Simpson, 13 1/2 years old, is in the hospital for treatment of newly diagnosed diabetes mellitus. A teaching program for Amy and her mother has been instituted by the nursing staff.

8. To plan a teaching program for Amy, the nurse should consider that the factor that will have the GREATEST influence on its success is

   A. the child's age
   B. the child's parents' acceptance of the diagnosis
   C. whether or not teaching is done consistently by the same nurse
   D. whether or not teaching is limited to one-hour periods

9. When teaching Amy and her parents about insulin, it is important to include the fact that insulin

   A. requirements will decrease with age
   B. dosage is determined, primarily, on the basis of daily food intake
   C. dosage, after adolescence, can be adjusted by the person in terms of variations in physical activity
   D. will be needed for life

10. One morning when the nurse goes to help Amy with morning care, Amy is argumentative and restless. She makes unkind remarks to the other children.
    It is essential for the nurse to give IMMEDIATE consideration to which of these questions?

    A. Does Amy need a more structured plan of care?
    B. When did Amy have her insulin and did she eat her breakfast?
    C. Was there some incident that occurred the previous day that has upset Amy?
    D. Is Amy bored and does she need help in selecting recreational activities that will utilize her excess energy?

10.____

11. One day Amy asks the nurse, *Will I be able to go with the gang after school to get ice cream or a hot dog?* Which of these responses by the nurse would give Amy accurate information?

    A. You can go with the group, but the hot dogs, ice cream, and other foods that they eat are prohibited for you. Your friends will learn to be considerate of your special needs.
    B. Both hot dogs and ice cream contain valuable nutrients. But if you have a hot dog, don't eat the roll.
    C. You can have a hot dog if you omit a corresponding amount of food from your next meal. Since sweets are not good for you, avoid foods like ice cream.
    D. Being with your friends is important. You can eat a hot dog or ice cream sometimes. We'll help you learn how to choose foods.

11.____

12. One day Amy tells her mother and the nurse that she does not want to give herself insulin. Her mother says to her, *You don't have to give yourself the injection if you don't want to. I'll do it for you.*
    Which of these understandings should be the basis of the nurse's response?

    A. The mother must be helped to understand the importance of the girl's participation in her own care.
    B. The girl needs to assume responsibility for her treatment; therefore, Amy and her mother should be taught separately.
    C. Children with diabetes often rebel against puncturing themselves with needles, and teaching should be discontinued until signs of readiness are demonstrated.
    D. The reaction of the mother is normal and should be overlooked.

12.____

13. A few days before Amy is discharged, her scout leader visits her. The scout leader stops at the nurses' station before leaving and says, *The troop is going on a four-day camping trip next month. Amy is very eager to go, and I'd like to have her come. But I'm rather concerned about having her out in the woods with us.*
    Before replying, which of these questions should the nurse consider?

    A. Are such trips contraindicated for children who have diabetes?
    B. Would it be too hazardous for Amy to attempt the trip so soon after her hospitalization?
    C. Will there be an adult accompanying the children who has had experience with children who have diabetes?
    D. Does Amy have enough information about her condition so that she is unlikely to have any difficulty?

13.____

14. Ms. Simpson says to the nurse, *Amy has never been a complainer. I'm afraid that she will not tell me if she doesn't feel well before she goes to school.* Which of these responses by the nurse would be MOST helpful to Amy's mother?

    A. It will be important to find out how Amy is feeling without stressing symptoms in talking with her.
    B. It is the school nurse's responsibility to help you with problems like this.
    C. Since Amy behaves this way, it will be necessary for you to question her frequently about how she feels.
    D. You don't need to worry about this because when Amy leaves the hospital her diabetes will be controlled.

15. In the management of a child with diabetes mellitus, occasional minimal glycosuria may be allowed.
    The purpose of this management is to

    A. retard degenerative tissue changes
    B. detect early symptoms of impending coma
    C. reduce the incidence of insulin shock
    D. facilitate diet supervision

Questions 16-22.

DIRECTIONS: Questions 16 through 22 are to be answered on the basis of the following information.

Jimmy Brown, 6 years old, is brought to the hospital immediately after sustaining burns that occurred in his home when he pulled a pan of boiling water off the stove. He has severe burns, mostly third degree, of the anterior chest, upper arms, forearms, and hands.

Jimmy is placed in a single room. An intravenous infusion is started, an indwelling urethral (Foley) catheter is inserted, and pressure dressings are applied to his burned areas.

16. Jimmy develops burn shock.
    He can be expected to exhibit

    A. restlessness and bradycardia
    B. air hunger and hyperreflexia
    C. intense pain and convulsions
    D. pale, clammy skin and thirst

17. To plan for Jimmy's fluid replacement needs, it should be noted that the

    A. younger the child, the greater amount of fluid he needs in proportion to his body weight
    B. proportion of body weight contributed by water is smaller during early childhood than it is during adulthood
    C. fluid needs per kilogram of body weight are variable until the kidneys become functionally mature at adolescence
    D. total volume of extracellular fluid per kilogram of body weight increases gradually from birth to adolescence and then stabilizes at the adult level

18. On admission, Jimmy's rectal temperature was 99° F. (37.2° C.) Twelve hours later, it is 101.6° F. (38.7° C.). On the basis of the information provided about him, it is MOST justified to say that it

   A. is an expected development in injuries such as Jimmy's
   B. is indicative of damage to Jimmy's heat-control center
   C. is a manifestation of rapidly spreading infection
   D. has resulted chiefly from a marked increase in serum potassium

18._____

19. Twenty-four hours after his admission, Jimmy complains that his chest dressing feels too tight.
    The nurse should FIRST

   A. check Jimmy's respirations
   B. loosen the chest bandage
   C. call the doctor
   D. find out whether Jimmy has a p.r.n. order for an analgesic

19._____

20. When selecting a site for the administration of a parenteral drug to Jimmy, it would be MOST important for the nurse to consider that

   A. impaired circulation hampers drug absorption
   B. decreased blood volume shortens the period of drug action
   C. drug action is potentiated by increased amounts of circulating epinephrine
   D. concentration of blood plasma in the tissues potentiates the desired effects of drugs

20._____

21. Which of these meals for Jimmy would be HIGHEST in proteins and calories?

   A. Vegetable soup, cottage cheese on crackers, applesauce, hot chocolate
   B. Cheeseburger, french fried potatoes, carrot sticks, cantaloupe balls, milk
   C. Fresh fruit plate with sherbet, buttered muffin, slice of watermelon, fruit-flavored milk drink
   D. Chicken noodle soup, cream cheese and jelly sandwich, buttered whole kernel corn, orange sherbet, cola drink

21._____

22. Jimmy is scheduled to go to the physical therapy department at 9:30 A.M. every day. One morning at 8:30, after Jimmy has had his breakfast, the nurse who goes in to bathe him finds him sound asleep.
    Which of these actions by the nurse would demonstrate the BEST judgment?

   A. Allow Jimmy to sleep until necessary equipment for his bath is gathered and then wake him for the procedure.
   B. Let Jimmy sleep and postpone his bath until sometime later in the day.
   C. Wake Jimmy gently and bathe him, explaining to him that he can rest when he returns from physical therapy
   D. Bathe Jimmy as quickly as possible and then let him sleep until it is time to go for physical therapy.

22._____

Questions 23-24.

DIRECTIONS: Questions 23 through 24 are to be answered on the basis of the following information.

Ralph Dunn, 15 years old, is admitted to the hospital for treatment of ulcerative colitis.

23. Ralph is receiving methantheline (Banthine) bromide. The CHIEF purpose of this drug for Ralph is to

   A. suppress inflammation of the bowel
   B. reduce peristaltic activity
   C. neutralize acid in the gastrointestinal tract
   D. increase bowel tone

24. Ralph is on a low-residue, high-protein, high-calorie diet.
   To meet the requirements of Ralph's diet prescription, the nurse should guide Ralph to select as an evening snack

   A. a roast beef sandwich
   B. strawberry shortcake with whipped cream
   C. canned peaches
   D. fresh orange juice

25. The nurse is discussing nutrition with the mother of two sons, a preadolescent and an adolescent. The mother should be instructed that in terms of nutritional needs, as compared with most normal preadolescent boys, MOST normal adolescent boys need _____ calories _____ protein.

   A. more; but less
   B. more; and more
   C. fewer; but more
   D. fewer; and less

KEY (CORRECT AHSWERS)

1. B		11. D	
2. A		12. A	
3. B		13. C	
4. D		14. A	
5. D		15. C	
6. D		16. D	
7. C		17. A	
8. B		18. A	
9. D		19. A	
10. B		20. A	

21. B
22. B
23. B
24. A
25. B

EXAMINATION SECTION
TEST 1

DIRECTIONS: Each question or incomplete statement is followed by several suggested answers or completions. Select the one that BEST answers the question or completes the statement. *PRINT THE LETTER OF THE CORRECT ANSWER IN THE SPACE AT THE RIGHT.*

1. Which approach by the nurse to a newly admitted toddler, who is not acutely ill, and to his mother would probably be MOST reassuring to both?

    A. Getting acquainted with the toddler before discussing his likes and dislikes with the mother
    B. Having the mother hold the toddler while questioning her about his habits
    C. Leaving the toddler with the play lady in the playroom while talking with the mother about his habits and preferences
    D. Holding the toddler while asking the mother questions about his habits

2. The nurse is assessing whether a normal 5-year-old is achieving the primary developmental task for children of his age.
   If the child is achieving this task, the child's behavior should indicate that he is developing a sense of

    A. trust   B. identity   C. intimacy   D. initiative

3. The mother of a 1-year-old and a 3-year-old is talking with the nurse about the eating habits of her children. In comparing the eating habits of most normal children of those ages, which DIFFERENCE is likely to be evident?

    A. The food intake of a 3-year-old will be about three times greater than that of a 1-year-old.
    B. A 1-year-old will have stronger food preferences than a 3-year-old.
    C. A 3-year-old will do more fingering of foods than a 1-year-old.
    D. The appetite of a 3-year-old is likely to be more capricious than that of a 1-year-old.

Questions 4-7.

DIRECTIONS: Questions 4 through 7 are to be answered on the basis of the following information.

Liz Thomas, 18 months old, is admitted to the hospital with symptoms of a subdural hematoma.

4. Liz's mother asks about her daughter's diagnosis. She should be told that a subdural hematoma is

    A. under the outer layer of the meninges
    B. between the inner layer of the meninges and the brain
    C. in the soft tissues of the scalp
    D. under the periosteum and above the meninges

5. Liz has a craniotomy with removal of a hematoma. Her condition is good. Mr. and Ms. Thomas are suspected of physically abusing Liz.
   The day after Liz's surgery, a nurse's aide says to the nurse, *Every time I see Ms. Thomas, I see red. How could any adult, least of all a mother, deliberately hurt a little child?*
   Which of these initial responses by the nurse would probably be MOST helpful to the aide?

   A. Making judgments about parents' actions is not appropriate for nursing personnel.
   B. You must not let Ms. Thomas know how you feel.
   C. It is an upsetting situation, isn't it?
   D. There is no legal proof that Liz's parents have been abusing her.

6. Which of these measures is MORE important for toddlers who have been battered than for other hospitalized toddlers?

   A. Providing opportunities for physical activity
   B. Arranging to have them cared for consistently by the same personnel
   C. Scheduling specific visiting times for parents
   D. Providing opportunities for play with other toddlers

7. A staff nurse asks the nurse in charge, *Suppose I report to the appropriate agency that a child in my community has sustained a multiplicity of unexplained injuries and may have been abused by the parents. What could happen to me for reporting this information?*
   If the state in which the nurse lives has a child abuse law that covers nurses, it would be CORRECT to say that he/she will be

   A. legally liable if a suit for slander is brought by the child's parents
   B. immune from legal action as a consequence of making the report
   C. exempt from appearing in court in defense of the child if a suit develops
   D. none of the above

Questions 8-11.

DIRECTIONS: Questions 8 through 11 are to be answered on the basis of the following information.

Gary Pott, 6 months old, is brought to the clinic by his mother. Gary has phenylketonuria and is on a phenylalanine-controlled diet.

8. The nurse encourages Ms. Pott to keep Gary on the prescribed diet.
   The nurse should include in her teaching plan the understanding that phenylketonuria is thought to be the result of

   A. insufficient fat intake during early infancy
   B. deficiency of an enzyme needed to utilize galactose during early infancy
   C. inability of the infant to metabolize one of the essential amino acids
   D. abnormal accumulation of lipids in the cells of infants

9. Ms. Pott should be instructed that the food that is HIGHEST in phenylalanine is

   A. fruits   B. fats   C. breads   D. jams

10. Ms. Pott tells the nurse that although her husband is working, his salary is small and they are having difficulty covering the cost of Gary's special feedings, along with other expenses.
Which of these actions would BEST exemplify the CORRECT role of the nurse in this situation?

   A. Help Ms. Pott to reassess her budget.
   B. Refer Ms. Pott to the doctor.
   C. Make an appointment for Ms. Pott with the social worker.
   D. Report Ms. Pott's problem to the local department of welfare.

11. All of the following descriptions of Gary's behavior are typical of a normal 6-month-old infant EXCEPT that he

   A. raises himself to a sitting position, but he cannot lie down without help
   B. babbles, but the babbling is not in response to a specific situation
   C. can hold a small object simultaneously in each hand, but he drops one or both of them after a short period
   D. bends his fingers to grasp an object, but he does not use a pincer motion to pick up an object

Questions 12-16.

DIRECTIONS: Questions 12 through 16 are to be answered on the basis of the following information.

One-month-old Susan Black is brought to the well child unit by her mother for her first clinic visit.

12. To assess the adequacy of an infant's weight, the MOST important index is the

   A. age at which the infant doubles his birth weight
   B. relationship between the infant's increase in height and weight
   C. infant's total weight gain since birth
   D. pattern of the infant's weight gain

13. Ms. Black tells the nurse that she gives Susan twice the prescribed amount of a multivitamin preparation because the prescribed amount seems so small.
The nurse's response should MOST certainly include the fact that

   A. it is uneconomical to give vitamins in excess of body requirements
   B. an infant's growth rate can be accelerated by vitamins in excess of the recommended daily requirements
   C. metabolic processes are stimulated by large amounts of vitamins
   D. excessive amounts of fat-soluble vitamins can be toxic

14. Examination reveals a possible congenital dislocation of Susan's left hip.
Which of these observations of an infant would be an early symptom of unilateral congenital dislocation of the hip?

   A. Flexion of the leg on the affected side and extension of the other leg when in the supine position
   B. Absence of a gluteal fold on the affected side

C. Limited abduction of the hip on the affected side
D. Prominence of the hip on the unaffected side

15. Susan is referred to an orthopedic clinic, and a diagnosis of congenital dislocation of the left hip is established. A splint that holds Susan's legs in frog position is used in her initial care.
    When Susan is 10 months old, she is admitted to the hospital; and, with closed manipulation, the head of her left femur is placed in the acetabulum. A hip spica cast is then applied. The cast extends from her waistline to below the knee on the left side and to a point above the knee on the right side.
    Which of these measures would probably be MOST helpful in preventing Susan from becoming unresponsive and withdrawn while she is hospitalized?

    A. Placing her in a room with several other infants the same age as she is
    B. Providing her with a variety of toys that she can handle
    C. Arranging for her mother to help with her care each day
    D. Keeping her regimen of care the same each day

16. If treatment for unilateral congenital dislocation of the hip had been delayed for Susan until after she walked, she would have been LIKELY to develop

    A. scoliosis and scissors gait
    B. pigeon toes and knock-knees
    C. a limp and lordosis
    D. waddling gait and knock-knees

Questions 17-25.

DIRECTIONS: Questions 17 through 25 are to be answered on the basis of the following information.

Mr. Ted Wynn, 17 years old, awakens one night because he is having difficulty breathing and noticeable wheezing on expiration. He is admitted to the hospital. He has a history of asthmatic attacks. His orders include isoproterenol (Isuprel) hydrochloride. Pulmonary function studies and other diagnostic tests will be done after his acute episode subsides.

17. The nurse should observe Mr. Wynn for

    A. pallor and dyspnea
    B. bradycardia and diplopia
    C. diarrhea and elevated blood pressure
    D. tachycardia and headache

18. All of the following information is provided by Mr. Wynn. The provoking factor of his asthmatic attack is probably that he

    A. wore a new suit made of a synthetic material two days ago
    B. smoked more cigarettes than usual during the past week
    C. has been up date at night playing cards with his friends
    D. slept on a new feather pillow

19. During the night, Mr. Wynn perspires profusely. The nurse should

    A. inform the physician
    B. watch him for signs of hypovolemic shock
    C. cover him with another blanket
    D. change his gown and sheets as needed

20. The MAJOR purpose of pulmonary function tests for Mr. Wynn is to

    A. determine his exercise tolerance
    B. determine which areas of his lungs are affected
    C. evaluate the extent of his ventilatory deficiency
    D. evaluate the adequacy of his cardio-pulmonary circulation

21. The next morning, Mr. Wynn has an acute asthmatic attack. Epinenphrine hydrochloride (Adrenalin) is administered to him.
    The nurse should observe Mr. Wynn for vasoconstricting effects of Adrenalin, which include

    A. drowsiness and hypotension
    B. throbbing headache and tremor
    C. flushed face and increase in body temperature
    D. polyuria and urticaria

22. During the asthmatic attack, Mr. Wynn spontaneously assumes an upright sitting position, which

    A. relieves the intrapleural pressure on the diaphragm
    B. stimulates the pleural reflex
    C. increases the muscle tone of the bronchioles
    D. permits a more efficient use of the muscles of respiration

23. All of the following measures should be carried out during Mr. Wynn's asthmatic episode EXCEPT

    A. keeping his environment quiet
    B. offering him sips of water
    C. teaching him how to deep-breathe and cough
    D. noting the amount and characteristics of his sputum

24. Mr. Wynn had all of the following diseases during his childhood. Which one may have had a relationship to his present illness?

    A. Rheumatic fever   B. Otitis media
    C. Chickenpox   D. Eczema

25. A desensitization program is prescribed for Mr. Wynn. He should be informed that the outcome of the program is usually MOST dependent upon the

    A. patient's age
    B. patient's response to antihistamines
    C. patient's ability to develop blocking antibodies
    D. type of serum used for the patient

KEY (CORRECT ANSWERS)

1. B
2. D
3. D
4. A
5. C

6. B
7. B
8. C
9. C
10. C

11. A
12. D
13. D
14. C
15. C

16. C
17. D
18. D
19. D
20. C

21. B
22. D
23. C
24. D
25. C

TEST 2

DIRECTIONS: Each question or incomplete statement is followed by several suggested answers or completions. Select the one that BEST answers the question or completes the statement. *PRINT THE LETTER OF THE CORRECT ANSWER IN THE SPACE AT THE RIGHT.*

1. The following four children completed their primary tetanus immunization 2 years ago. Which child would be MOST likely to receive a booster dose of toxoid now?

    A. Bill, who sustained several long scratches on his bare legs while climbing on a backyard fence
    B. Sue, who is hospitalized and having emergency treatment for a perforated appendix
    C. John, who is having dental treatment for an abscessed impacted molar
    D. Amy, who walked barefoot around a vacation ranch and cut her foot on a broken bottle

    1.____

2. The eating habits of most healthy young adolescents probably BEST reflect their need to

    A. conform to peer behavior
    B. look like a favorite adult
    C. spend short periods at a variety of activities
    D. have new experiences

    2.____

3. A mother calls a neighbor who is a nurse and says that her toddler ate an unknown plant in the backyard and now appears ill.
   In addition to telling the mother to call a doctor immediately, which of the following advice would it be APPROPRIATE for the nurse to give the woman?

    A. Obtain a urine specimen from the child.
    B. Have the child drink an ounce of mineral oil.
    C. Put the child to bed and elevate his extremities.
    D. Make the child vomit and save the vomitus.

    3.____

4. The CHIEF difficulty in establishing a therapeutic relationship with most children who are autistic stems from the fact that they

    A. have a functional hearing defect
    B. are mentally retarded as well as mentally ill
    C. behave in a manner difficult to understand
    D. are unable to follow directions

    4.____

5. Which of these measures is the MOST important one to consider in the home management of a young child who is mentally retarded?

    A. Having the same person teach him all new activities
    B. Limiting the amount of stimulation he receives from his environment
    C. Maintaining a consistent routine for the performance of his activities of daily living
    D. Teaching him amenities that will help him to be accepted by others

    5.____

6. An infant has erythroblastosis fetalis (hemolytic disease of the newborn). The parents should be informed that the development of jaundice in the infant is caused by

   A. an overproduction of erythrocytes
   B. an abnormal production of melanin
   C. excessive destruction of red blood cells
   D. hypobilirubinemia

7. A child with an eye infection is to have physiologic saline eye irrigations. When carrying out an eye irrigation, it is CORRECT to

   A. use a solution in which there is a tablespoon of salt in each quart of water
   B. use only enough pressure to maintain a steady flow of solution along the lower conjunctival sac
   C. direct the flow of solution toward the inner surface of the upper lid
   D. keep the head flat

Questions 8-14.

DIRECTIONS: Questions 8 through 14 are to be answered on the basis of the following information.

Lisa Smith, 2 years old, is admitted to the hospital with acute otitis media of the right ear. Her body temperature is elevated.

8. Lisa's susceptibility to otitis media is due to the fact that the

   A. eustachian tube is short and wide in children
   B. causitive organism is part of the normal flora in throats of children
   C. external ear in children is less effective in resisting the entrance of foreign objects
   D. inner ear in children is markedly immature

9. Lisa is to have a tepid sponge bath. To achieve the desired outcome of this procedure, the nurse should

   A. stroke Lisa's skin to cause friction
   B. give Lisa warm fluids to drink
   C. allow moisture on Lisa's skin to evaporate
   D. lower the temperature of Lisa's room

10. Lisa has severe pain in her right ear. The pain of acute otitis media is due CHIEFLY to

    A. reduced tension on structures in the vestibular portion of the inner ear
    B. constriction of the endolymphatic spaces in the labyrinth of the inner ear
    C. increased pressure of fluid in the middle ear
    D. irritation of the stapes in the middle ear

11. Lisa is to receive 100,000 U. of an oral suspension of penicillin four times a day. A bottle containing 300,000 U. of penicillin in 5 cc. of solution is to be used to prepare Lisa's dosage.
How much solution will contain the amount of penicillin prescribed for Lisa?
_____ cc.

    A. 0.7   B. 1.7   C. 2.7   D. 3.7

12. Lisa's condition improves.
Ms. Smith says to the nurse, *I need to go home to see how my mother is making out with my other children; but each time I try to leave, Lisa gets so upset that I just can't,*
Which of these responses by the nurse would probably be BEST?

    A. Lisa is now well enough to be without you. Why don't you try slipping away when she falls asleep?
    B. Stress is not good for Lisa even though her condition is improved. Is it possible for you to find out about the children without leaving Lisa?
    C. Your feeling torn about whether to stay or go is understandable when Lisa needs you too. Whenever you're ready to go, let me know and I'll stay with her.
    D. Lisa needs to be more independent of you now. Your being away from her for a while will help her.

13. Lisa has a temper tantrum one morning while her mother is bathing her. Ms. Smith asks the nurse how the behavior should be handled.
In replying, the nurse should include that this behavior in 2-year-olds

    A. indicates regression
    B. suggests a poorly developed sense of trust
    C. should be controlled by parental discipline
    D. is a normal outlet for tension

14. A member of the nursing team remarks to the team leader,
Lisa whines and fusses all the time her mother is with her. She quiets down as soon as she leaves but cries when she comes back. I wonder if it's good for her to visit so often.
Which of these responses would probably help the team member MOST to think through the problem?

    A. This is a characteristic trait of children this age. Haven't you noticed it in others?
    B. This behavior may be indicative of a disturbed mother-child relationship. You should continue to watch them closely.
    C. Even if the mother upsets the child, she should be encouraged to continue to visit as often as she can.
    D. Is it possible that her mother's being with her enables her to express her unhappiness?

Questions 15-21.

DIRECTIONS: Questions 15 through 21 are to be answered on the basis of the following information.

When 16-month-old Ann Wolfe is admitted to the hospital, she has a temperature of 104° F. (40° C.), petechiae, and purpuric areas on her skin. A diagnosis of meningococcal meningitis is established.

15. Ann has opisthotonos.
    Which of these positions will be BEST for her while she has this symptom?

    A. Semi-Flowler's
    B. Side-lying
    C. Dorsal recumbent
    D. Prone

16. While Ann is acutely ill, which of these measures will be ESSENTIAL in her care?

    A. Reducing environmental stimuli
    B. Maintaining optimum nutrition
    C. Preventing the development of herpetic lesions of the lips
    D. Exercising her extremities passively several times a day

17. Ann is being watched for signs of adrenal insufficiency. Which of these symptoms are characteristic of this condition?
    _____ blood pressure and _____.

    A. Normal; increasing pulse rate
    B. Rising; weak, thready pulse
    C. Falling; weak, thready pulse
    D. Fluctuating; decreasing pulse rate

18. Ann is receiving both an antibiotic and a sulfonamide. Because she is receiving a sulfonamide, which of these daily measures will be ESPECIALLY important for her?

    A. Weighing her and observing her for edema
    B. Giving her extra fluids and measuring her fluid intake and output
    C. Taking her blood pressure and her apical pulse at regular, specified intervals
    D. Observing her frequently for signs of photophobia and hyperreflexia

19. A spinal tap is done to assess Ann's response to therapy. Which change in Ann's spinal fluid would be indicative of improvement in her condition?

    A. *Increase* in cell count
    B. *Increase* in specific gravity
    C. *Decrease* in sugar
    D. *Decrease* in protein

20. Ann responds favorably to treatment and is convalescing. In order to meet Ann's nutritional needs, her food plan should be based on which of these needs of normal 16-month-old children?

    A. Their diets should include a variety of foods that they can eat by themselves.
    B. Liquids and semiliquids are best for them.
    C. Preference should be given to their favorite foods.
    D. Milk is of greater importance to them than solids.

21. After Ann recovers, which type of immunity to the meningococcus will she have?

    A. Passive acquired
    B. Cellular
    C. Natural
    D. Active acquired

Questions 22-24.

DIRECTIONS: Questions 22 through 24 are to be answered on the basis of the following information.

Suzanne Edwards, 6 years old, is admitted to the hospital for probable repair of a ventricular septal defect. This is Suzanne's third hospital admission.

22. Suzanne has a cardiac catheterization.
    For the first few hours after the cardiac catheterization, which of these nursing measures will be ESSENTIAL for her?

    A. Keeping the head of her bed elevated 30 degrees
    B. Encouraging her to cough forcefully at regular intervals
    C. Checking her temperature every hour
    D. Taking her pulse frequently in the extremity used for the cutdown

22.____

23. In preparing Suzanne for the proposed surgery, which characteristic of 6-year-old children should be given GREATEST consideration by the nurse?

    A. Concrete experiences are most meaningful.
    B. The ability to think abstractly is well-developed.
    C. Cause and effect relationships are readily understood.
    D. The ability to distinguish between fantasy and reality is well-developed.

23.____

24. Suzanne has open-heart surgery for repair of a ventricular septal defect. She is then transferred to the intensive care unit.
    During Suzanne's surgery, her femoral arteries were cannulated.
    As a result of this procedure, it is ESSENTIAL postoperatively for the nurse to make frequent checks of Suzanne's

    A. urinary output
    B. pedal pulses
    C. rectal temperature
    D. ability to move her lower extremities

24.____

25. A woman phones a nurse at home and says that her son fell and broke his eyeglasses and that she thinks some glass may have penetrated one eye.
    The nurse advises immediate medical attention and that in the meanwhile it would be MOST important for the mother to

    A. apply a pressure dressing to the affected eye and keep the child in an erect sitting position
    B. examine the affected eye to determine whether any glass can be easily removed and apply petrolatum (Vaseline) on the outer surface of the eyelid
    C. loosely cover both eyes and have the child remain quiet
    D. gently irrigate the affected eye with a copious aount of boiled table salt solution that has cooled and leave the eye uncovered

25.____

KEY (CORRECT ANSWERS)

1. D
2. A
3. D
4. C
5. C

6. C
7. B
8. A
9. C
10. C

11. B
12. C
13. D
14. D
15. B

16. A
17. C
18. B
19. D
20. A

21. D
22. D
23. A
24. B
25. C

TEST 3

DIRECTIONS: Each question or incomplete statement is followed by several suggested answers or completions. Select the one that BEST answers the question or completes the statement. *PRINT THE LETTER OF THE CORRECT ANSWER IN THE SPACE AT THE RIGHT.*

1. When a primipara's normal first-born infant is brought to her for the first feeding, she says, *He's so little! I'm afraid I'll hurt him.*
   Which of these responses would be MOST helpful from the standpoint of learning?

   A. You can practice taking care of the baby while you're here.
   B. Is there someone at home who can help you with the baby the first few weeks?
   C. You can watch me take care of the baby.
   D. The public health nurse can come to your home to show you how to take care of the baby.

1.____

Questions 2-4.

DIRECTIONS: Questions 2 through 4 are to be answered on the basis of the following information.

Ms. Marie DuPont, who was discharged two days ago from the post-partum unit, is visiting her newborn girl on the pediatric unit. Baby girl DuPont has a cleft lip and cleft palate.

2. The nurse should expect that because Ms. DuPont has an infant with an obvious physical defect, Ms. DuPont may

   A. have difficulty loving such an infant and responding warmly to it
   B. overtly express love for the infant because mother love is instinctive
   C. express mixed feelings for the infant that will require psychiatric treatment to overcome
   D. express guilt that will require her visits with the infant to be curtailed

2.____

3. Ms. DuPont is concerned about the likelihood of having other children with the same anomaly as her baby girl's. Ms. DuPont should be given which of the following information about her probability of having another child with a cleft palate?

   A. If this mother has close medical supervision during subsequent pregnancies, the anomaly is not likely to occur again.
   B. Since the anomaly is so rare, it is highly unlikely that a mother would have more than one child with such an anomaly.
   C. There is little probability that future children of this mother will have the same anomaly since there is no genetic basis for its development.
   D. A mother's having one child with this anomaly means that there is a greater-than-average possibility of her having other children with the same anomaly.

3.____

4. Children with cleft palates are MOST likely to have

   A. abnormal dentition, speech impairments, and recurrent otitis media
   B. inadequate nutrition, poor muscle coordination, and mental retardation
   C. persistent infantile emotional pattern, regression in speech development, and hearing deficit
   D. accelerated caries formation, peer group maladjustment, and maternal overprotection

4.____

Questions 5-10.

DIRECTIONS: Questions 5 through 10 are to be answered on the basis of the following information.

John Stone, a 3 1/2-year-old, was admitted to the hospital because of a persistent bleeding from a minor laceration. His condition is diagnosed as classic hemophilia (factor VIII deficiency).

5. Because of John's age, which of these aspects of hospitalization is likely to be MOST traumatic for him?

    A. Being inhibited from running about freely
    B. Being separated from his family
    C. Being placed in an unfamiliar environment
    D. Having his routines and rituals disrupted

6. John is an only child. His parents are concerned about the possibility of their future offspring having hemophilia.
   His parents should be told that

    A. male offspring will have the hemophilic trait and will either be carriers or will have the bleeding tendency; female offspring will not be subject to the condition
    B. hemophilia is unlikely to occur in female offspring, but they can be carriers; male offspring have a 50 percent chance of having the condition
    C. the probability that hemophilia will occur in other offspring is no greater than it is in the general population
    D. each of their offspring will have a 25 percent chance of having hemophilia, a 50 percent chance of being a carrier, and a 25 percent chance of being free of the gene for hemophilia

7. Before his illness, John had achieved all of the following abilities.
   Which ability did he probably develop MOST recently?

    A. Throwing a large ball four to five feet
    B. Putting a spoon in his mouth without spilling the contents
    C. Speaking in sentences of three or four words
    D. Alternating his feet while walking upstairs

8. All of these measures should be considered in feeding John.
   Which one is MOST important in terms of the development needs of a 3 1/2-year-old?

    A. Using colorful child-size cups and dishes for his food
    B. Having him sit at a table that is of a height appropriate for his size
    C. Serving him small portions of food
    D. Letting him feed himself

9. In discussing dental prophylaxis for John with Mr. and Mrs. Stone, the nurse should tell them that dental visits should be

    A. scheduled only when definite symptoms occur
    B. preceded by the administration of antihemophilic globulin (AHG) factor VIII
    C. scheduled at regular intervals
    D. started when the deciduous teeth become loose

10. Which of these understandings about John should his parents be helped to gain?

    A. John's participation in active range-of-motion activities will help to prevent contractures.
    B. John's emotional development will be fostered by a warm, indulgent family, but some curtailment of his physical development may result.
    C. Overprotection may impede John's emotional and physical development.
    D. Children with John's condition tend to limit their own physical activity.

Questions 11-18.

DIRECTIONS: Questions 11 through 18 are to be answered on the basis of the following information.

Ms. Wendy Stevens, 18 years old, is admitted to the hospital with a diagnosis of infectious hepatitis (Type A). Her orders include bed rest and diagnostic studies.

11. On admission, Ms. Stevens should be expected to have which of these early symptoms of infectious hepatitis (Type A)?

    A. Loss of appetite
    B. Ecchymoses
    C. Shortness of breath on exertion
    D. Abdominal distension

12. Which of these factors in Ms. Stevens' history is MOST likely to be related to her diagnosis?

    A. Recent recovery from an upper respiratory infection
    B. Being bitten by an insect
    C. Contact with a person who was jaundiced
    D. Eating home-canned foods

13. The nurse should monitor the results of which of these tests that is used to assess Ms. Stevens' liver function?

    A. Serum transaminase   B. Protein-bound iodine
    C. Creatinine clearance   D. Glucose tolerance

14. All of the following precautionary measures are essential in Ms. Stevens' case EXCEPT

    A. serving food on disposable dishes
    B. wearing a face mask
    C. carrying out procedures for decontamination of urine and feces
    D. modifying procedures for discarding used syringes and needles

15. The CHIEF purpose of bed rest for Ms. Stevens is to

   A. minimize liver damage
   B. reduce the breakdown of fats for metabolic needs
   C. decrease the circulatory load to reduce cardiac effort
   D. control the spread of the disease

16. Members of Ms. Stevens' family who have been exposed to infectious hepatitis should be given

   A. penicillin
   B. sulfadiazine
   C. immune human serum globulin
   D. irradiated plasma

17. Ms. Stevens' condition improves.
   The nurse is planning Ms. Stevens' care during her convalescent period.
   The nurse should expect that Ms. Stevens will have the MOST difficulty with

   A. relieving pain
   B. regulating bowel elimination
   C. maintaining morale
   D. preventing respiratory complications

18. As a result of her having hepatitis, Ms. Stevens should be instructed NEVER to

   A. smoke
   B. eat fried foods
   C. donate blood
   D. exercise strenuously

Questions 19-25.

DIRECTIONS: Questions 19 through 25 are to be answered on the basis of the following information.

Alison Wright, 19 months old, is diagnosed by the family doctor as having acute laryngotracheobronchitis. Alison's temperature is 103° F. (39.4° C.) when Ms. Wright brings her to the hospital. This is Alison's first hospital admission.

19. Two early symptoms that are MOST likely to occur in laryngotracheobronchitis are

   A. cough and inspiratory stridor
   B. elevated temperature and prostration
   C. Kussmaul respirations and bradycardia
   D. flushed face and labored expirations

20. Ms. Wright tells the nurse, who is filling out a habit record for Alison, that Alison has achieved bowel control. Which additional information would it be MOST important for the nurse to obtain from Ms. Wright at this time?

   A. The extent of Ms. Wright's understanding of the regressive effect of illness and hospitalization on bowel-training in children of Alison's age
   B. Alison's toileting routines at home
   C. The age at which Alison's bowel-training was started
   D. Whether Alison has indicated readiness for bladder-training

21. Alison is placed in a Croupette.
    Restraints are to be used on Alison because she continually tries to get out of the Croupette. Because Alison requires the restraints, the nurse should

    A. tell Alison's mother that bilateral arm and leg restraints are necessary for toddlers
    B. inform Alison's mother that Alison will probably adjust better to restraints if she is left alone for a while after they are applied
    C. explain to Alison the need for the restraints in order to help her adjust to them
    D. watch Alison carefully after the restraints are applied to see whether she struggles to the point of negating the value of the therapy

    21.____

22. Which of these symptoms in Alison could give the EARLIEST indication of increased respiratory difficulty?

    A. Generalized cyanosis
    B. Increased pulse rate
    C. Decreased respiratory rate
    D. Abdominal breathing

    22.____

23. Alison is to receive a dose of aspirin in liquid form. In view of her condition and her age, it would be BEST to

    A. support Alison in a sitting position, hold the medicine glass with the medication to her lips, and tell her calmly and firmly to drink it
    B. turn Alison on her side, give her a straw, and tell her to suck the medication from the medicine glass
    C. hand Alison the medicine glass containing the drug and tell her to drink it, saying that it will taste like candy
    D. mix the medication in a 4-ounce glass of sweetened fruit juice, prop Alison up in a sitting position, give her the glass, and tell her in a positive tone to drink the juice

    23.____

24. Alison's condition improves, and the Croupette is discontinued. Diet as tolerated is ordered for her.
    A nurse's aide reports to the nurse that although Alison seems hungry, she pushes the aide's hand away and will not eat when the aide tries to feed her. The nurse should communicate to the aide that most children of Alison's age

    A. eat better when seated at a table with adults
    B. prefer to feed themselves
    C. have finicky appetites
    D. have strong food preferences

    24.____

25. A normal 19-month-old child can be expected to

    A. stand briefly on one foot without support and to put together simple jigsaw puzzles
    B. drink through a straw and to know his own sex
    C. manage finger foods and to understand *No, no*
    D. build a tower of 7 blocks and to open doors by turning knobs

    25.____

KEY (CORRECT ANSWERS)

1.	A	11.	A
2.	A	12.	C
3.	D	13.	A
4.	A	14.	B
5.	B	15.	A
6.	B	16.	C
7.	D	17.	C
8.	D	18.	C
9.	C	19.	A
10.	C	20.	B

21. D
22. B
23. A
24. B
25. C

EXAMINATION SECTION
TEST 1

DIRECTIONS: Each question or incomplete statement is followed by several suggested answers or completions. Select the one that BEST answers the question or completes the statement. *PRINT THE LETTER OF THE CORRECT ANSWER IN THE SPACE AT THE RIGHT.*

Questions 1-9.

DIRECTIONS: Questions 1 through 9 are to be answered on the basis of the following information.

Mr. and Mrs. Smitts bring their 3 1/2-year-old son, Jimmy, to the hospital emergency room at 2 A.M. They state that he awoke with noisy respirations and a barking cough. The physician makes a diagnosis of laryngotracheobronchitis (croup) and admits Jimmy to the hospital.

1. While admitting Jimmy, the nurse might observe

   A. expiratory wheezing
   B. a decreased pulse
   C. inspiratory stridor
   D. a temperature of 103° F

2. Mrs. Smitts is present during Jimmy's admission to the pediatric unit and she remains in a corner of the room. When the nurse speaks to her, she answers in a quivering voice. To decrease Mrs. Smitts' anxiety, the nurse should encourage her to

   A. discuss her fears concerning Jimmy's illness
   B. wait in the waiting room
   C. answer questions about Jimmy's health history
   D. assist in taking Jimmy's pulse

3. Jimmy is placed in a mist tent to ease his respiration. He starts calling for his parents and pulling on the canopy in a struggle to get out of the tent.
   The FIRST thing that the nurse should do is

   A. administer the medication to sedate Jimmy
   B. give Jimmy a bottle of milk or juice to help him fall asleep
   C. explain to Jimmy about the mist tent and remain with him until he is no longer crying
   D. put clove hitch restraints on Jimmy to restrict him from pulling on the mist tent

4. Jimmy's respiratory rate remains higher than normal. The nurse should notify the physician IMMEDIATELY if she observes

   A. substernal retractions
   B. emesis of undigested food
   C. restlessness followed by severe fatigue
   D. flaring nostrils with each inspiration

5. Because of increasing respiratory distress, Jimmy goes through a tracheostomy.
   An IMPORTANT intervention for Jimmy's nursing care plan is to

A. administer chest physiotherapy every 3 hours
B. suction Jimmy's tracheostomy every 12 hours
C. change Jimmy's dressing every day
D. have a hemostat available at the bedside all the time

6. The nurse is MOST likely to decrease Jimmy's anxiety before his tracheostomy is suctioned by telling him:

   A. After I clean your tube, you can go to the playroom
   B. I must clean your tube in order for you to get better soon
   C. Here is your car to play with while I am cleaning your tube
   D. You are such a good little boy; I know that you won't move

7. While Jimmy has his tracheostomy and is still in the mist tent, of the following, the MOST appropriate toy for him is

   A. a beanbag
   B. plastic nesting blocks
   C. a musical doll
   D. a coloring book

8. Jimmy has had his tracheostomy plugged and is now on a regular diet. His mother is assisting him with lunch. Mrs. Smitts tells the nurse that Jimmy's appetite is poor compared to what it was during infancy.
The BEST reply by the nurse to Mrs. Smitts would be:

   A. You need not be concerned; most children of Jimmy's age have a poor appetite
   B. You should ask your pediatrician to prescribe vitamins for Jimmy
   C. Jimmy's appetite will improve as soon as he returns home
   D. Jimmy's growth rate is now slower, thus it is normal for his appetite to decrease

9. While planning for discharge, Mrs. Smitts expresses her fear about Jimmy's experiencing another severe upper respiratory infection in the future. She asks the nurse what to do if this occurs.
The MOST appropriate response by the nurse would be:

   A. Take Jimmy into the bathroom and turn on a hot shower
   B. Teaching appropriate breathing exercises to Jimmy can prevent any further attacks
   C. Give Jimmy a lot of fluids in order to liquefy his secretions
   D. Call your local emergency squad immediately

Questions 10-15.

DIRECTIONS: Questions 10 through 15 are to be answered on the basis of the following information.

Luisa Tate's first child was delivered 10 hours ago. She is about to breastfeed her infant for the first time since his initial feeding on the delivery table.

10. The nurse discusses the lengths of feedings with Mrs. Tate before she starts feeding her infant.
The MOST appropriate time schedule would be

   A. as long as the infant is willing
   B. until Mrs. Tate starts feeling soreness in her breasts

C. 4 minutes on each breast the first day, 6 minutes the second day, 8 minutes the third day, and 10 to 15 minutes on each breast thereafter
D. 4 minutes on each breast the first day and 10 minutes on each breast thereafter

11. When Mrs. Tate feeds her baby for the first time, the nurse should

    A. leave the room so Mrs. Tate can interact with her infant
    B. assist Mrs. Tate to start the feeding and then leave so that she can interact with her infant, checking back at intervals on how they are doing
    C. take the baby from Mrs. Tate at intervals to burp him
    D. remain at the bedside throughout the feeding

12. While assisting Mrs. Tate in breastfeeding her infant, the nurse tells her to place the brown pigmented area around the nipple well into the baby's mouth.
    The reason for this is to

    A. make the infant feel more secure
    B. minimize breast engorgement
    C. promote erection of the nipple
    D. improve the efficiency of the baby's sucking

13. Mrs. Tate experiences *afterpains* when she nurses her baby. She asks the nurse whether she needs to stop nursing because of this.
    The nurse's BEST response would be:

    A. This will disappear in a few days, so you can postpone nursing until then
    B. Pain is not a serious complaint, so there is no reason to stop
    C. This is rather an unusual complaint, so it would be best for you to stop nursing
    D. Nursing stimulates the uterus to contract and helps it return to its normal size. You should not stop nursing, but I can give you medication if you are too uncomfortable.

14. Mrs. Tate asks the nurse about how to adjust her diet while she is breastfeeding.
    The breastfeeding mother needs an average of _____ additional calories daily.

    A. 2500   B. 1500   C. 1000   D. 500

15. Mrs. Tate is concerned about her baby getting germs from her while breastfeeding.
    The MOST important measure she should be taught to prevent bacterial contamination of the baby is

    A. not allowing anyone in the room while she breastfeeds her baby
    B. washing her hands before each feeding
    C. wearing sterile pads inside her bra
    D. cleansing her nipples with an antiseptic solution each day

Questions 16-25.

DIRECTIONS: Questions 16 through 25 are to be answered on the basis of the following information.

Four-year-old George Harrison is admitted to the pediatric unit with a tentative diagnosis of acute lymphoblastic leukemia. He has a history of frequent respiratory tract infections, accompanied by a low-grade temperature and fatigue. George seems to be very anxious and pale.

16. At the time of admission, which of the following procedures will George fear the MOST?

    A. Obtaining his weight and height
    B. Assessing his pulse and respirations
    C. Collecting a urine specimen
    D. Taking his temperature rectally

17. The primary nurse prepares a nursing care plan for George.
    On the basis of George's history, the nurse would write the following nursing diagnosis.
    Potential for infection related to

    A. a decreased production of erythrocytes
    B. an invasion of bone marrow by leukemic cells
    C. an increased production of immature lymphocytes
    D. enlargement of the spleen, liver, and lymph nodes

18. During the assessment of George's skin, the nurse finds petechie and multiple ecchymotic areas on his extremities. The nurse adds the following nursing diagnosis to George's care plan.
    Potential for injury related to a(n)

    A. decrease in hemoglobin
    B. decrease in platelet formation
    C. iron deficiency
    D. abnormality in the clotting mechanism

19. The physician needs to perform a bone marrow aspiration on George's posterior iliac crest.
    After this procedure,

    A. the site of the bone marrow aspiration must be observed for bleeding
    B. vital signs will be taken every 10 minutes for two hours
    C. George must remain flat in his bed for 45 minutes
    D. the nursing care plan does not require revision

20. The physician decides to place George on L-asparaginase. Which of the following describes the action of this medication?

    A. Nucleic acid synthesis is interfered with by disrupting folic acid metabolism.
    B. Leukemic cells are destroyed by preventing the incorporation of an essential amino acid needed for protein synthesis.
    C. Cell reproduction is interfered with by blocking the incorporation of purine into nucleic acids.
    D. The metabolic breakdown of xanthine to uric acid is prevented.

21. George is also receiving vincristine.
    The nurse observes George for potential side effects of this medication, including

    A. hemorrhagic cystitis, mucosal ulceration, and infertility
    B. anorexia, stomatitis, and hepatic dysfunction

C. neurotoxicity, alopecia, and constipation
D. nephrotoxicity, diarrhea, and dermatitis

22. George is receiving a transfusion of packed cells. He complains of a sharp pain and chills in his back. The nurse notes his vital signs and finds that George's respirations and pulse are above normal and that he has an elevated temperature.
The MOST appropriate intervention by the nurse at this time would be to

    A. slow down the transfusion and administer an anti-histamine
    B. stop the transfusion, send a sample of George's urine to the laboratory, and notify the physician
    C. slow down the transfusion and assess George's vital signs every 20 minutes
    D. stop the transfusion, place George in a semi-Fowler's position, and notify the head nurse

22.____

23. The nurse taking care of George observes that his gums are bleeding.
The BEST intervention for the nurse to utilize when providing George with mouth care would be to

    A. have George brush his teeth frequently, using a stiff toothbrush
    B. encourage George to rinse his mouth with a sodium bicarbonate solution after each meal
    C. allow George to perform oral cleansing in the same manner as he does at home
    D. swab George's mouth frequently with cotton swabs moistened with half-strength hydrogen peroxide

23.____

24. The nurse is administering morning care to George. George wants to assist her.
Which of the following tasks can be performed by George himself without assistance?

    A. Take his bath
    B. Brush his teeth
    C. Completely dress himself
    D. Undress himself

24.____

25. George is on bedrest.
Of the following activities, the MOST appropriate one for George at this time is

    A. playing with a running train
    B. drawing a picture about his stay in the hospital
    C. playing checkers with a boy his age
    D. watching television

25.____

KEY (CORRECT ANSWERS)

1. C
2. A
3. C
4. C
5. D

6. B
7. B
8. D
9. A
10. C

11. B
12. D
13. D
14. C
15. B

16. D
17. C
18. B
19. A
20. B

21. C
22. B
23. D
24. D
25. B

TEST 2

DIRECTIONS: Each question or incomplete statement is followed by several suggested answers or completions. Select the one that BEST answers the question or completes the statement. *PRINT THE LETTER OF THE CORRECT ANSWER IN THE SPACE AT THE RIGHT.*

Questions 1-6.

DIRECTIONS: Questions 1 through 6 are to be answered on the basis of the following information.

Six-month-old Peter Dunhill is brought to the hospital because he has had five to six watery green stools every day for the last 3 days. After being checked by a pediatrician, he is admitted to the pediatric unit with a diagnosis of gastroenteritis.

1. The head nurse should assign Peter to a   1.____

    A. two-bedded room currently occupied by an eight-month-old infant with bronchitis
    B. private room, located next to the utility room
    C. two-bedded room, currently occupied by a two-month-old infant with pyloric stenosis
    D. private room, with a sink, located across from the nurses' station

2. The pediatrician notices that Peter has mild isotonic dehydration.   2.____
   The BEST method for the nurse to observe Peter's level of dehydration each scheduled time is to

    A. measure intake and output
    B. assess his skin turgor
    C. determine his weight
    D. palpate his anterior fontanelle

3. Peter is placed on NPO and IV therapy is instituted. The nurse taking care of Peter   3.____
   notices that 500 cc of fluid has run in during the last hour.
   The MOST appropriate intervention by the nurse would be to

    A. discontinue the IV therapy and notify the intravenous therapist
    B. decrease the rate of flow, take the apical pulse, and notify the pediatrician
    C. stop the IV flow, assess the blood pressure, and notify the head nurse
    D. regulate the rate of flow to the correct amount, assess for signs of dehydration, and notify the head nurse

4. Prolonged diarrhea in children can lead to acid-base imbalance.   4.____
   The nurse taking care of Peter should assess him often for

    A. deep and rapid respirations
    B. a rapid and thready pulse
    C. slow and shallow respirations
    D. an elevation in blood pressure

5. Assessment of Peter's skin reveals excoriation of the buttocks.
   The MOST appropriate nursing intervention to facilitate healing would be to cleanse the excoriated area

   A. and give a heat lamp treatment for 20 minutes
   B. with baby body lotion and put on clean diapers
   C. apply Desitin ointment and expose the buttocks to air for a few minutes
   D. with soap and water and apply baby powder

6. Peter's condition is now improved, and his IV therapy is stopped. His pediatrician gradually resumes solid foods. A soft food that would be APPROPRIATE for Peter at this time is

   A. oatmeal
   B. plain yogurt
   C. pureed apples
   D. custard

Questions 7-12.

DIRECTIONS: Questions 7 through 12 are to be answered on the basis of the following information.
Baby George Brown is 10 hours old. His parents started the bonding process with him in the delivery room and are now seeing him for the second time.

7. The Browns seem worried because the baby's head appears elongated.
   The nurse's BEST reply about the cause of elongated head would be

   A. a genetically inherited trait
   B. the overlapping of bones during birth
   C. a collection of blood under the bones
   D. a collection of fluid under the tissues

8. Baby George passes his first stool while he is with his parents. They are startled by its appearance, but the nurse tells them that it is a normal first stool.
   The first stool of a newborn is

   A. yellow, soft, and well-formed
   B. greenish yellow and soft
   C. brownish and putty-like in appearance
   D. blackish green, thick, and sticky

9. The Browns ask why the baby jumped when the crib was bumped.
   The nurse tells them that it is a normal neurological response known as the _____ reflex.

   A. rooting
   B. Babinski
   C. Moro
   D. tonic neck

10. Of the following, the reflex that may indicate an abnormality in a newborn is a _____ reflex.

    A. one-sided Moro
    B. positive rooting
    C. positive grasp
    D. positive Babinski

11. The nursery nurse does a complete newborn assessment on baby George. While inspecting the infant's fontanelles, which of the following observations would suggest an abnormality? 11.____

    A. Anterior fontanelle diamond-shaped
    B. Bulging anterior fontanelle
    C. Posterior fontanelle smaller than anterior
    D. Posterior fontanelle difficult to palpate

12. Baby George should be watched carefully for signs of infection if Mrs. Brown has a history of 12.____

    A. Pitocin use during labor
    B. a urinary tract infection during her third trimester
    C. membranes ruptured prior to 24 hours before delivery
    D. an episode of bleeding during the second trimester

Questions 13-17.

DIRECTIONS: Questions 13 through 17 are to be answered on the basis of the following information.

During a screening program for lead poisoning run by a child health clinic in an inner city community, it is discovered that 32-month-old Linda Loveless has an elevated blood lead level. She and her family live in a rundown two-family house. Her mother says that Linda has been very irritable lately and has a poor appetite. She is admitted to the pediatric unit of the local hospital for further treatment.

13. The MOST likely cause of lead poisoning in children of Linda's age group is 13.____

    A. eating paint and plaster chips
    B. eating vegetables sprayed with insecticide
    C. inhaling fumes from a local chemical factory
    D. playing with toys decorated by lead-based paint

14. The initial nursing assessment reveals that Linda gets tired easily, has a poor appetite, is pale, and is irritable. 14.____
    The diagnosis that would be MOST correct to be formulated by the nurse on the basis of the given data is

    A. potential alteration in growth and development secondary to lead toxicity
    B. potential for injury related to lead in the environment
    C. alteration in tissue perfusion, cerebral, secondary to lead toxicity
    D. alteration in tissue perfusion related to interference with hemoglobin synthesis secondary to lead toxicity

15. Linda is going to be treated with intramuscular injections of EDTA and BAL. 15.____
    The nurse taking care of Linda thinks, of the following interventions, the HIGHEST priority should be

    A. changing the injection sites
    B. allowing the child to hold the syringe

C. applying warm soaks to the injection sites
D. giving sitz baths after administering injections

16. Linda should be assessed by the nurse, after having received the chelating agent, for side effects, including

    A. nephrotoxicity
    B. neurotoxicity
    C. gastrointestinal distress
    D. immunosuppression

17. Linda's blood lead level has returned to normal, and she is now ready to be discharged. During the discharge planning, the nurse advises Mrs. Loveless to

    A. observe Linda for signs of developmental delays
    B. have Linda's blood lead level checked every 3 months
    C. prevent Linda from putting nonedible objects into her mouth
    D. move from her present apartment as soon as possible

Questions 18-25.

DIRECTIONS: Questions 18 through 25 are to be answered on the basis of the following information.

Eight-year-old Sonya Cory is admitted to the pediatric unit with a tentative diagnosis of rheumatic fever. She has a fever of 101.5° F and a fine pink rash on her trunk. She also complains of pain in her knees and ankles.

18. The nurse attending Sonya and her mother during the admission procedure asks whether Sonya has had any recent infections.
    Which of the following statements by Sonya's mother reflects the USUAL pattern in children diagnosed with rheumatic fever?
    Sonya

    A. has not had any infections recently
    B. had impetigo 2 months ago
    C. had a sore throat 3 weeks ago
    D. complained of a sore throat 3 days ago

19. The nurse assessing Sonya observes for the major manifestations of rheumatic fever. These include

    A. anemia, temperature, and carditis
    B. subcutaneous nodules, polyarthritis, and carditis
    C. arthralgia, epistaxis, and erythema marginatum
    D. arthralgia, chorea, and elevated temperature

20. Sonya's physician decides she should be on complete bed-rest. The PRIMARY rationale for this intervention is to

    A. decrease the workload on Sonya's heart
    B. prevent severe damage to Sonya's joints

C. prevent the spread of the streptococcal infection
D. prevent chorea manifestations

21. One of the highest nursing priorities is to assess Sonya for signs of carditis. The clinical manifestation MOST likely to be present if Sonya suffers carditis is a(n)

    A. elevated blood pressure
    B. elevated sleeping pulse
    C. widening pulse pressure
    D. slow and thready pulse

22. Sonya is placed on aspirin, grain XX, every 6 hours. The signs of toxicity in this case would include

    A. dermatitis and anemia
    B. projectile vomiting and diarrhea
    C. tinnitus and hyperpnea
    D. blurring of vision and increased blood pressure

23. Sonya still feels pain in her knees and ankles. The BEST nursing intervention to make Sonya more comfortable would be

    A. putting ice packs on the involved joints
    B. starting a program of passive and active motion exercises
    C. placing a bed cradle on the bed and positioning Sonya in the proper anatomical alignment
    D. massaging the involved joints with warm normal saline soaks

24. Of the following activities, the one that would be the MOST appropriate for Sonya while she is on bedrest is

    A. cutting out paper dolls with an eight-year-old girl suffering of pneumonia
    B. playing checkers with a ten-year-old girl who has a fractured forearm
    C. making potholders with a nurse's aide
    D. playing cards with a nine-year-old girl suffering of juvenile rheumatoid arthritis

25. During the discharge planning discussion, which of the following statements by Mrs. Cory indicates the need for further guidance by the nurse?

    A. Sonya should walk eight blocks to school each day.
    B. Sonya shares a small bedroom with her two sisters.
    C. Our family lives in a second-floor walk-up apartment.
    D. Sonya's younger brother had a tonsillectomy three weeks ago.

KEY (CORRECT ANSWERS)

1. D
2. C
3. B
4. A
5. A

6. B
7. B
8. D
9. C
10. A

11. B
12. C
13. A
14. D
15. A

16. A
17. C
18. C
19. B
20. A

21. B
22. C
23. C
24. B
25. B

EXAMINATION SECTION
TEST 1

DIRECTIONS: Each question or incomplete statement is followed by several suggested answers or completions. Select the one that BEST answers the question or completes the statement. *PRINT THE LETTER OF THE CORRECT ANSWER IN THE SPACE AT THE RIGHT.*

Questions 1-9.

DIRECTIONS: Questions 1 through 9 are to be answered on the basis of the following information.

Ms. Evelyn Hart, a 75-year-old widow, is admitted to a psychiatric hospital. Her son, who brings her, says that she has been confused and wandered away from home. Also, she has become increasingly careless about her appearance.

1. With a chronic brain syndrome such as Ms. Hart's, the personality changes are MOST often manifested as.

    A. an exaggeration of previous traits
    B. overt pleas for assistance
    C. suspicion and reticence
    D. marked resistance and negativism

2. During the early period following Ms. Hart's admission, the nursing procedure that would be BEST for her is

    A. carrying out activities in the same order each day
    B. insisting that she focus her conversation on present events
    C. providing a variety of novel experiences
    D. rotating staff assignments so that she will become acquainted with each member of the nursing staff

3. When Ms. Hart's son comes to visit her the day after admission, Ms. Hart refuses to talk to him. The son goes to the nurse and says, *My mother won't talk to me. Why is she acting like this? I had to do something with her. I couldn't keep her with us. Oh, what a mess!* Which of these responses by the nurse would be MOST appropriate initially?

    A. You feel guilty about having your mother here.
    B. Your mother is having a little difficulty adjusting to the hospital.
    C. This is a difficult situation for you and your mother.
    D. I'm sure you did the best you could under the circumstances.

4. Ms. Hart's son asks the nurse whether he should come to see his mother again on the following day in view of her reaction to his first visit.
Which of these responses would be BEST?

    A. Advising the son to wait until his mother gives some indication that she is ready to see him
    B. Suggesting that the son come back the next day since his continuing interest is important to his mother

C. Telling the son that his mother will not miss him if he doesn't visit because she will become attached to staff members
D. Informing the son that it is important for his mother to have visitors and suggesting that he ask one of her friends to visit her

5. The nurse finds Ms. Hart standing near the lavatory door. She has wet herself - as she does occasionally - because she does not allow herself sufficient time to reach the bathroom. Ms. Hart looks ashamed and turns her head away from the nurse.
Which of these responses by the nurse would be BEST?

    A. Asking, *Can you tell me why you wait so long, Ms. Hart?*
    B. Saying, *I know that this is upsetting to you, Ms. Hart. Come with me and I'll get a change of clothes for you*
    C. Asking, *Can you think of any way in which we can help you to manage your bathroom trips, Ms. Hart?*
    D. Sending Ms. Hart to her room to change her clothing

6. At about 3 P.M. one day, Ms. Hart comes to the nurse and says, *I haven't had a thing to eat all day.* The nurse knows that Ms. Hart did have lunch.
Which of these understandings by the nurse should be BASIC to a response?

    A. Confabulation is used by elderly patients as a means of relieving anxiety.
    B. Hunger is symbolic of a feeling of deprivation.
    C. Retrospective falsification is a mechanism commonly used by elderly persons who are unhappy.
    D. Loss of memory for recent events is characteristic of patients with senile dementia.

7. Ms. Hart is to be encouraged to increase her intake of protein.
The addition of which of these foods to 100 cc. of milk will provide the GREATEST amount of protein?

    A. 50 cc. light cream and 2 tablespoons corn syrup
    B. 30 grams powdered skim milk and 1 egg
    C. 1 small scoop (90 grams) vanilla ice cream and 1 tablespoon chocolate syrup
    D. 2 egg yolks and 1 tablespoon sugar

8. One day when another patient, Mr. Simon, is about to go to the canteen, Ms. Hart says to him, *Bring me a candy bar.* Mr. Simon replies, *Okay, give me the twenty-five cents for it.* Ms. Hart struggles with the idea, taking out a quarter and holding it but not giving it to Mr. Simon. Mr. Simon goes off impatiently, and Ms. Hart looks forlorn.
Which of these responses by the nurse would probably be MOST useful to Ms. Hart?

    A. *Ms. Hart, when we get things from the canteen, we have to pay for them. Do you want to buy candy?*
    B. *It was hard for you to decide whether or not to give Mr. Simon the money for the candy. Let's go to the canteen together.*
    C. *I know you are upset about Mr. Simon's going off, but he did have a right to ask you for the money for the candy.*
    D. *You feel you annoyed Mr. Simon. Would you like to talk about it?*

9. Ms. Hart tells stories over and over about her childhood. One day she keeps talking about holidays and how she used to make cookies for visiting children.
Which of the responses by the nurse would be BEST?

   A. That must have been a lot of fun, Ms. Hart. Will you help us make popcorn balls for the unit party?
   B. I can understand that those things were important to you, Ms. Hart. Now we can talk about something that is going on in the unit.
   C. Things are different now, Ms. Hart. What does your family serve as party refreshments nowadays?
   D. Those were the good old days. Did you ever go on a hayride?

Questions 10-17.

DIRECTIONS: Questions 10 through 17 are to be answered on the basis of the following information.

Mr. David Tripp, 28 years old, is brought from his place of work to the emergency department of a local general hospital by the police. He had been threatening his supervisor, who had criticized his work. During the admission procedure, he says, *They're all in on the plot to lock me up so I can't protect the world from them.*

10. During the early period of Mr. Tripp's hospitalization, which of these plans of care would probably be BEST for him?

    A. Encourage him to enter into simple group activities.
    B. Establish a daily routine that will help him become oriented to this new environment.
    C. Plan to cope with his slowness in carrying out his daily schedule.
    D. Assign the same members of the nursing team to care for him each day.

11. Mr. Tripp is on chlorpromazine hydrochloride (Thorazine) 100 mg. t.i.d. and 200 mg. at h.s.
The CHIEF purpose of chlorpromazine for Mr. Tripp is to

    A. relieve his anxiety
    B. control his aggression
    C. decrease his psychotic symptoms
    D. alleviate his depression

12. Mr. Tripp is walking into the dayroom when a male patient runs toward him screaming, *Let me out! Let me out!* A nurse's aide is following the screaming patient and is talking soothingly to him. Mr. Tripp seems panic-stricken and turns to flee.
Which of these initial responses to Mr. Tripp by the nurse would be BEST?

    A. Don't go, Mr. Tripp. That patient won't hurt you. He is frightened.
    B. It is upsetting to hear someone scream. The aide will help that patient. I will stay with you for a while, Mr. Tripp.
    C. Don't be upset, Mr. Tripp. That patient is sicker than you are. It's all right for you to go to your room if you like.
    D. This is nothing to be disturbed about, Mr. Tripp. It is part of that patient's illness.

13. One afternoon, Mr. Tripp is sitting in a small lounge watching a TV news program. During a biographical sketch of a criminal, Mr. Tripp begins to shout frantically, No, I am not one! You've no right to say that! Mr. Tripp's response to the program is MOST clearly an example of

   A. an idea of reference
   B. an obsession
   C. confabulation
   D. negativism

14. Mr. Tripp seems to value his regular sessions with the nurse, but on one occasion he becomes agitated and suddenly gets up and starts to mumble and pace back and forth. Which of these actions by the nurse would be BEST when Mr. Tripp does this?

   A. Sit quietly, while remaining attentive to him.
   B. Join him and pace with him.
   C. Leave the room until he calms down.
   D. Get a male nurse's aide to come and stand by and observe Mr. Tripp.

15. Mr. Tripp, who has read widely in the field of psychology, quotes fluently from various authorities with whose works the nurse is only vaguely acquainted.
   Which of these actions by the nurse in this situation would probably be BEST?

   A. Make an attempt to learn more about psychology in order to be able to converse with Mr. Tripp.
   B. Point out to Mr. Tripp that such theoretical knowledge is of little value unless it is applied in daily life.
   C. Listen attentively, in a relaxed manner, without attempting to compete with Mr. Tripp.
   D. Ask Mr. Tripp if he understands why he feels the need to give evidence of his knowledge of psychology.

16. Mr. Tripp is much improved and is to go home for a weekend. Since he is taking chlorpromazine hydrochloride (Thorazine), he should be given information regarding side-effects such as

   A. loss of pubic hair and weight gain
   B. agranulocytosis and nausea
   C. gastrointestinal bleeding and gynecomastia
   D. susceptibility to sunburn and potentation of alcohol

17. One day Mr. Tripp remarks to the nurse, Now that I can concentrate move, I can probably hold down a job when I'm discharged from the hospital.
   Which of these responses by the nurse would probably be MOST appropriate?

   A. Don't you expect to go back to your old job, Mr. Tripp?
   B. You have improved, Mr. Tripp, but you must be careful not to take on too much.
   C. Have you thought of something you might like to do, Mr. Tripp?
   D. There are agencies that will find work for you when you are ready, Mr. Tripp.

Questions 18-25.

DIRECTIONS: Questions 18 through 25 are to be answered on the basis of the following information.

Ms. Nancy Balm, a 20-year-old former music student, is admitted to a psychiatric hospital. Six months after entering school, she was dismissed for engaging in drug parties and sexual orgies in the dormitory. She has also been involved in the theft of a car and in several minor traffic violations. Ms. Balm has grown up in a permissive atmosphere with few controls.

18. After a few days, it is noted that Ms. Balm frequently seeks the attention of one of the female nurses; Ms. Balm calls her by her first name, offers to help her with her work, and frequently tells her that she is the nicest person on the unit.
Based on Ms. Balm's history, it is probably MOST justifiable to say that she

   A. has developed the capacity to be concerned about other people
   B. is asking for help from this nurse
   C. is attempting to use this nurse for her own purposes
   D. genuinely likes this nurse

18.____

19. Ms. Balm is on a locked unit. A new nurse on the unit is about to leave and is holding the key. Ms. Balm approaches, saying eagerly, *Let me turn the key and unlock the door. The other nurses let me.*
Which response by the nurse would be MOST appropriate?

   A. Going to the nurse in charge to ask if Ms. Balm's request should be granted
   B. Telling Ms. Balm in a friendly way that this is not permissible
   C. Letting Ms. Balm turn the key in the lock but keeping close to her while she does it
   D. Asking Ms. Balm why she feels that it is important for her to turn the key

19.____

20. One day Ms. Balm talks with the nurse about the events that led up to her hospitalization. She volunteers the information that she had stolen a car.
Considering the kind of illness she has, which additional comment that she might make would probably BEST indicate her basic attitude?

   A. I wanted a new sportscar, and that one was just what I had been looking for, so I took it.
   B. For a long time, I had wanted to steal a car but had been able to control my desire, but finally it overpowered me.
   C. I knew it was wrong to steal a car, but my friend dared me to.
   D. Once I had driven away in the car, I was sorry I had taken it.

20.____

21. At unit parties, Ms. Balm frequently dances with an elderly man who has chronic brain syndrome. She is courteous to him, though somewhat condescending. The elderly patient receives the attention happily.
It would be CORRECT for staff members to make which of these evaluations about this situation?

   A. Ms. Balm should not be permitted to dance with the elderly patient.
   B. Personnel should let Ms. Balm know that they are aware she is using this means to get approval.
   C. The elderly patient will terminate their relationship if he ceases to obtain pleasure from it.
   D. The activity need not be interrupted as long as both Ms. Balm and the elderly patient receive satisfaction from it.

21.____

22. A young male nurse who works with Ms. Balm has been going to the unit in the evening to see her. When questioned about this, the nurse states that he is fond of Ms. Balm.
It would be ESSENTIAL for the nurse to recognize that

    A. his emotional involvement with Ms. Balm may interfere with his therapeutic effectiveness
    B. Ms. Balm's emotional involvement with him may interfere with her progress
    C. hospital policy prohibits romantic relationships between patients and nurses
    D. Ms. Balm may prove so demanding that he will drop the relationship, thus traumatizing her

23. When Ms. Balm's parents come to see her, they berate her for disgracing them, but they demand special privileges for her from the staff.
It is probably MOST justified to say that they

    A. are unable to express their love directly to their daughter
    B. feel protective toward their daughter
    C. feel that a permissive environment would be better for their daughter
    D. have conflicting feelings about their daughter

24. Several patients are in the dayroom singing with a piano accompaniment. Ms. Balm enters and interrupts the group by turning on the television set. In addition to turning off the television set, which of these responses by the nurse would be MOST appropriate?

    A. Ask Ms. Balm if she would like to lead the group singing.
    B. Tell Ms. Balm that she cannot use the television while the group is singing and offer her a choice of some other activities.
    C. Tell Ms. Balm that she can watch television later.
    D. Tell Ms. Balm that she cannot stay in the dayroom if she continues to disturb the group.

25. Several weeks after Ms. Balm's admission, a group of patients who have written a play for a hospital party ask her to read the script because they know she had a story printed in the hospital newspaper. Ms. Balm agrees to do so and makes several good suggestions to the group, but does not try to assume control of the project.
It is MOST justifiable to say that she is

    A. expressing a need to be liked
    B. indifferent to this project
    C. using a new method of manipulating the group
    D. showing improvement

KEY (CORRECT ANSWERS)

1.	A	11.	C
2.	A	12.	B
3.	C	13.	A
4.	B	14.	A
5.	B	15.	C
6.	D	16.	D
7.	B	17.	C
8.	B	18.	C
9.	A	19.	B
10.	D	20.	A

21. D
22. A
23. D
24. B
25. D

TEST 2

DIRECTIONS: Each question or incomplete statement is followed by several suggested answers or completions. Select the one that BEST answers the question or completes the statement. *PRINT THE LETTER OF THE CORRECT ANSWER IN THE SPACE AT THE RIGHT.*

Questions 1-9.

DIRECTIONS: Questions 1 through 9 are to be answered on the basis of the following information.

Andrew Miles, 18 years old and living away from home for the first time, is a freshman in college. He is admitted to the hospital because he has been having episodes in which he runs about, screams, and then drops to the floor and lies motionless for a few minutes, after which he gets up, mumbles *I'm sorry,* and behaves normally. His school record has been satisfactory, but his contacts with his peer group have decreased greatly because of these episodes. On the basis of diagnostic studies, it has been determined that Mr. Miles' illness is schizophrenia, catatonic type.

1. Stereotyped behavior such as that shown by Mr. Miles can be BEST explained as a(n)   1._____

    A. way of assuring predictability
    B. device to gain help and treatment
    C. means of increasing interpersonal distance
    D. attempt to control inner and outer forces

2. The behavior demonstrated by patients such as Mr. Miles is USUALLY thought to be indicative of   2._____

    A. damage to the cortex of the brain
    B. an expression of intrapersonal conflict
    C. a deficiency of vitamin B complex in the diet
    D. a disturbance in intellectual functioning

3. Upon Mr. Miles' admission, his needs would BEST be met by a plan that provides   3._____

    A. an introduction to each member of the staff
    B. a climate that makes few demands on him
    C. minimal sensory stimulation
    D. time for him to reflect on his problems without interference

4. The day after Mr. Miles' admission, a nurse, Ms. Caan, is assigned to stay with him for a period every day in order to establish a therapeutic nurse-patient relationship.   4._____
In carrying out this assignment, it is ESSENTIAL for this nurse to understand that Mr. Miles will probably

    A. be extremely sensitive to the feeling tones of others
    B. be unaware of the nurse's presence
    C. be hostile and verbally abusive
    D. talk if the nurse introduces topics that are of interest to him

5. Which of these insights that Mr. Miles might gain would be MOST basic to his improvement?

    A. Introjection of parental standards in childhood contributed to my personality.
    B. I am a person of worth and value.
    C. My behavior interferes with the development of good relationships.
    D. I require more reassurance than most people do.

6. One day a nurse finds Mr. Miles and another young male patient having an argument in the lounge. The other patient says, *Don't criticize me, you phony. You and your fits!* The other patient is pressing the argument, and Mr. Miles has run behind a chair.
   Which of these measures by the nurse would probably be BEST?

    A. Attempting to find out who started the argument
    B. Firmly directing each patient to go to his room
    C. Engaging the attention of the dominant patient
    D. Explaining to the other patient that Mr. Miles cannot control his spells

7. Mr. Miles now carries on brief conversations with Ms. Caan. During one such conversation, he seems relaxed and affable initially but soon begins to shift his position frequently, grasping the arms of his chair so tightly that his fingers blanch. Ms. Caan remarks to Mr. Miles that he seems tense, to which he replies *Yes*.
   Which of these responses by the nurse at this time would demonstrate the BEST understanding?

    A. I'm beginning to feel tense too, Mr. Miles.
    B. I wonder if I have said something wrong, Mr. Miles.
    C. Do women usually make you feel nervous, Mr. Miles.
    D. At what point in our talk did you begin to feel uneasy, Mr. Miles?

8. When Ms. Caan tells Mr. Miles that she will be off duty for two days, he says flatly, *So what. It doesn't matter.* It is MOST accurate to say that Mr. Miles is

    A. incapable of manifesting emotion
    B. confident of his ability to manage without the nurse
    C. controlling expression of his feelings
    D. apathetic toward the nurse

9. Family therapy is recommended for Mr. Miles. When explaining the purpose of this type of therapy to Mr. Miles' family, which of the following information would it be important to convey to them?

    A. Family members can reinforce the therapist's recommendations between sessions.
    B. Family members need advice in dealing with the identified patient's behavior.
    C. Joint treatment permits equal participation, eliminating anxieties that might otherwise lead to termination of treatment.
    D. Joint treatment alters family interaction, facilitating change in the behavior of the identified patient.

Questions 10-16.

DIRECTIONS: Questions 10 through 16 are to be answered on the basis of the following information.

Fifty-year-old Mr. Jack Dunn, accompanied by his wife, is brought to the emergency room by the police. He has been despondent because he was not promoted in his job. After calling his son to say goodbye, insisting that he was going to end it all, he locked himself in the bathroom, and the police were called to get him out. Mr. Dunn is admitted to the psychiatric unit.

10. Which of these interpretations of Mr. Dunn's behavior should serve as the basis for formulating his nursing care plan?
He

   A. wants to punish those around him
   B. is trying to manipulate his environment
   C. is attempting to get attention and sympathy
   D. is looking for relief from helplessness and hopelessness

10.____

11. Which of these statements ACCURATELY assesses Mr. Dunn's potential for suicide?
His

   A. sex and present stress suggest a high risk, but the likelihood of suicide is low in his age group
   B. threat suggests that the risk of suicide is minor
   C. age, sex, and present stress suggest a high risk of suicide
   D. sex suggests a low risk since suicide occurs 30 times more often in females than in males

11.____

12. Which of these occurrences would be MOST likely to result in an INCREASE in Mr. Dunn's suicidal thoughts?
His

   A. expressing hostility overtly before he is able to tolerate doing so
   B. entrance into a deeply retarded phase of depression
   C. being required to perform work in the kitchen
   D. being allowed to talk about his morbid ideas

12.____

13. During a staff conference concerning Mr. Dunn's care, a young nursing student says, *Even though I know that* Mr. Dunn's condition requires time to respond to therapy, I feel discouraged when I'm with him. No matter what I do, he talks about his failures and makes no attempt to help himself.
The interpretation of the student's reaction to Mr. Dunn's behavior that is probably MOST justifiable is that the

   A. student's difficulty arises from an attitude of hopelessness toward older persons
   B. student feels that Mr. Dunn's condition is not remediable unless he is willing to help himself
   C. student has set up a failure situation that is detrimental to therapeutic usefulness to Mr. Dunn
   D. student's self-concept as a helping person is being threatened

13.____

14. A nurse finds Mr. Dunn cutting his wrist with a razor blade.
Which of these actions should the nurse take?

   A. Shout *Stop!* and then say, *Tell me what caused your despair.*
   B. Say, *Think of what it would do to your family!*
   C. Grab Mr. Dunn's arm to stop him and say, *I'm going to stay with you.*
   D. Say, *Why, Mr. Dunn! You've just begun to feel better and now look what you've done.*

14.____

15. Mr. Dunn seems improved and is sent home on a trial visit. He is then admitted to the intensive care unit for treatment for a self-inflicted gunshot wound in the chest. When he is somewhat improved, Mr. Dunn remarks, *Everyone here must think I'm some kind of freak.*
Which of these responses would be MOST appropriate?

   A. None of us thinks that you are a freak.
   B. You feel that others are judging you.
   C. I understand that you were upset when this happened.
   D. What made you so desperate that you did a thing like this?

15.____

16. Mr. Dunn has improved and is discharged. A few days after Mr. Dunn returns to work, while he is talking with a co-worker, a number of things go wrong in the office. Mr. Dunn slams a book on the table and says, *Dammit!* The co-worker who is present is aware that Mr. Dunn has been mentally ill.
Which of these actions on the part of the co-worker would be BEST?

   A. Wait for Mr. Dunn to cool off and then resume the discussion.
   B. Suggest that Mr. Dunn go home and remain there until he calms down.
   C. Urge Mr. Dunn to take his tranquilizers.
   D. Talk with Mr. Dunn about his particular need for controlling outbursts.

16.____

Questions 17-25.

DIRECTIONS: Questions 17 through 25 are to be answered on the basis of the following information.

Ms. Julia Warren, 53 years old and with no previous history of mental illness, is admitted to a private psychiatric hospital because of symptoms, including pacing, wringing her hands, moaning, beating her forehead, and saying, *I'm a terrible woman.* She has been unable to do her job as a bookkeeper and has had to have members of her family stay with her day and night.

17. The extent of the nurse's orientation of Ms. Warren to the hospital environment should be based CHIEFLY upon Ms. Warren's

   A. willingness to stay with the nurse
   B. ability to concentrate
   C. persistence in making demands on other patients
   D. acceptance of the need for hospitalization

17.____

18. During the acute phase of Ms. Warren's illness, it is ESSENTIAL that the nurse have the ability to

    A. minimize stimuli in Ms. Warren's environment
    B. interest Ms. Warren in a variety of activities
    C. accept Ms. Warren's self-accusations
    D. strengthen Ms. Warren's intellectual defenses

19. Ms. Warren shows typical distress upon being informed of her impending electric convulsive therapy. Which understanding by the nurse would BEST serve as the basis for preparing Ms. Warren psychologically for it?

    A. Misinformation may be contributing to her anxiety.
    B. Emphasizing the safety of the procedure will reduce her fear.
    C. Knowing that most people have the same response is usually comforting.
    D. A high level of anxiety renders an individual more receptive to information given by helping persons.

20. Depressions of the type Ms. Warren has usually respond well to electric convulsive therapy, but the consequent memory loss is quite disturbing.
    The nurse can be MOST helpful to the patient who has such a loss of memory by

    A. engaging the patient in diversional activities
    B. reporting the problem to the physician
    C. explaining to the patient that other patients receiving this therapy also have this problem
    D. reassuring the patient repeatedly that this is an expected and temporary reaction

21. Which of the following defense mechanisms is MOST likely to be used by a person who is as depressed as Ms. Warren?

    A. Turning against the self
    B. Projection
    C. Rationalization
    D. Displacement of instinctual aims

22. When Ms. Warren learns that occupational therapy has been ordered for her, she scoffs at the idea, saying it is silly.
    If Ms. Warren were to think all of the following thoughts regarding occupational therapy, which one would be MOST acceptable to her?

    A. This is enjoyable.
    B. I'm helping to pay for my care.
    C. This keeps me from thinking about my failures.
    D. I didn't know that I was so creative.

23. Ms. Warren is assigned to group therapy. Which of these ideas would it be MOST desirable for each participant to gain?

    A. Each person's opinion is respected.
    B. Verbalization will help each individual to gain insight.
    C. Each member has a responsibility to other members of the group.
    D. The group work consists of analyzing each other's motivations.

24. Ms. Warren improves and goes out with her husband for the afternoon. That evening, a nurse finds Ms. Warren sitting by herself in the dayroom.
Which of these comments by the nurse would probably be BEST?

    A. Why are you so preoccupied, Ms. Warren?
    B. You look tired, Ms. Warren. Was your afternoon too much for you?
    C. You seem very quiet, Ms. Warren.
    D. You looked happier yesterday, Ms. Warren.

25. Ms. Warren is discharged. The day Ms. Warren goes back to work, Bob, a customer she has known for many years, comes in and says, *Hello there, Julia. Good to see you back! your boss told me that you were sick. What was wrong with you?* Which of these replies by Ms. Warren would indicate that she accepted her illness and has recovered?

    A. I was kind of mixed up for a while, Bob, but I'm all right now.
    B. I just didn't feel good, Bob. Old age coming on, I guess.
    C. I was just down in the dumps, Bob, but my doctor insisted that I go to the hospital. You know how they are.
    D. I'm glad to be back. What can I do for you, Bob?

KEY (CORRECT ANSWERS)

1.	D	11.	C
2.	B	12.	A
3.	B	13.	D
4.	A	14.	C
5.	B	15.	B
6.	C	16.	A
7.	D	17.	B
8.	C	18.	C
9.	D	19.	A
10.	D	20.	D

21.	A
22.	B
23.	A
24.	C
25.	A

TEST 3

DIRECTIONS: Each question or incomplete statement is followed by several suggested answers or completions. Select the one that BEST answers the question or completes the statement. *PRINT THE LETTER OF THE CORRECT ANSWER IN THE SPACE AT THE RIGHT.*

Questions 1-7.

DIRECTIONS: Questions 1 through 7 are to be answered on the basis of the following information.

When Mark Levine, 5 1/2 years old, goes to school for the first time, he screams and seems terrified when he sees the drinking fountain near his classroom door. Mark's mother tells the school nurse that he has an intense fear of drinking fountains.

1. The understanding of Mark's fear of fountains that is MOST justifiable is that it

   A. is a symptom common in dyslexic children
   B. is not subject to his conscious control
   C. stems from his lack of understanding of plumbing
   D. results from having learned that his symptoms have a manipulative potential

2. Behavior therapy will be used in treating Mark's symptoms. His plan of care will include

   A. authoritative instruction
   B. increased cultural orientation
   C. direct interpretations
   D. systematic desensitization

3. Mark's behavior reflects his need to control anxiety by

   A. refusing to recognize the source of his anxiety
   B. making a conscious effort to avoid situations that cause anxiety
   C. substituting a neutral object as the target of his negative feelings
   D. acting in a manner opposite to his underlying need

4. Parents should be instructed that a child's mental health will BEST be promoted if the love he receives from his parents

   A. is related to the child's behavior
   B. is unconditional
   C. makes externally imposed discipline unnecessary
   D. is reinforced by unchanging physical demonstrations

5. Ms. Levine calls the community mental health clinic and tells the nurse that Mark has suddenly become terrified of getting into the family car, refuses to do so, and is in the yard screaming uncontrollably.
   What would it be BEST for the nurse to tell Ms. Levine to do FIRST?

   A. Hold Mark snugly and talk softly to him.
   B. Give Mark a warm bath and put him to bed.
   C. Bring Mark to the clinic as soon as possible.
   D. Remind Mark that he has never before been afraid of automobiles.

6. Mark is having play therapy.
   The choice of play therapy for children of Mark's age should PROBABLY be based upon their inability to

   A. overcome inhibitors about revealing family conflicts and behaviors
   B. differentiate between reality and fantasy
   C. recognize the difference between right and wrong
   D. adequately describe feelings and experience

7. On a rainy day, after Mark's play-therapy session, Ms. Levine hands Mark his overshoes and says, *Put them on. It's pouring outside.* Mark answers defiantly, *No, they're too hard to put on. I can't.* Then he sits down on a bench and pouts. Ms. Levine looks at the nurse in a perplexed way, saying nothing.
   Which of these responses by the nurse would probably be BEST?

   A. Say to Ms. Levine, *Maybe the overshoes are too small to Mark.*
   B. Sit on the bench with Mark and say calmly, *It's raining. You start pulling your overshoes on, and I'll help you with the hard part.*
   C. Hand Mark his overshoes and say to him in a matter-of-fact way, *If you will put the first one one, I'll put on the second one for you.*
   D. Say to Mark, firmly but kindly, *You are trying to test your mother's authority. This behavior will not be tolerated. Put your overshoes on right now.*

Questions 8-14.

DIRECTIONS: Questions 8 through 14 are to be answered on the basis of the following information.

Ms. Eileen Gray, 33 years old, is admitted to the psychiatric hospital with a diagnosis of obsessive-compulsive reaction. Her chief fear is that her excreta may harm others on the unit. As a result, she spends hours in the bathroom washing not only her hands, arms, vulva, and anal area, but also the walls, toilet, and toilet stall. In the process, she discards wet paper towels in every direction and leaves puddles of water everywhere.

8. Ms. Gray's symptoms are MOST clearly an example of

   A. sublimation of anxiety-producing fantasies and daydreams
   B. compensation for an imaginary object loss
   C. a symbolic expression of conflict and guilt feelings
   D. an infantile maneuver to avoid intimacy

9. On the unit, Ms. Gray carries out her elaborate washing routine several times a day. She says to the nurse, *I guess all this seems awfully silly to you.*
   It is MOST justifiable to say that she

   A. is asking the nurse to keep her from performing these unreasonable acts
   B. really believes her acts are completely rational, and she is testing the nurse
   C. is indicating an appreciation of the unreasonable-ness of her behavior
   D. is deliberately putting the nurse in a difficult position

10. The nurse should understand that the probable effect of permitting Ms. Gray to perform her washing routines will be to

   A. confirm a basic delusion
   B. help Ms. Gray to perceive how illogical her behavior is
   C. create distrust of the nurse, who ought to symbolize reality
   D. temporarily reduce Ms. Gray's anxiety

11. Ms. Gray is unable to get to the dining room in time for breakfast because of her washing rituals.
    During the early period of her hospitalization, it would be MOST appropriate to

   A. wake Ms. Gray early enough so that she can perform her rituals in time to get to breakfast
   B. firmly insist that Ms. Gray interrupt her rituals at breakfast time
   C. explain to Ms. Gray that her rituals are not helping her to get well
   D. give Ms. Gray a choice between completing her rituals or going to breakfast

12. During a nursing team conference, staff members voice frustration concerning Ms. Gray's constant questions such as *Shall I go to lunch or finish cleaning my room?* and *Should I go to O.T. or mend my coat?*
    In order to deal effectively with this behavior, team members should know that Ms. Gray's

   A. dependence upon staff is a symptom that needs to be interrupted by firm limit-setting
   B. inability to make decisions reflects her basic anxiety about failure
   C. indecisiveness is meant to test the staff's acceptance of her
   D. relentless need to seek attention represents a developmental arrest at the autistic (prototaxic) level

13. Ms. Gray is being treated by psychotherapy. The physician tells the nurse to expect her to be upset at times when she returns from her session with him and to let her be upset.
    By this directive, the physician MOST probably wants to

   A. put Ms. Gray under stress so that she will become more responsive to suggestions
   B. teach Ms. Gray to be satisfied with advice from only one person
   C. help Ms. Gray become aware of her feelings
   D. make Ms. Gray independent, which would not be possible if she were to develop alliances with members of the nursing staff

14. Ms. Gray is given her first pass to spend the night at home. As the time approaches for her to leave the hospital, she seems increasingly tense and says, *Maybe I shouldn't stay home all night. Maybe I should just stay for dinner and then come back here.* When the nurse responds nondirectively, Ms. Gray answers, *I'm just sort of anxious about things in general. It's nothing specific.*
    Which of these responses by the nurse would probably be BEST?

   A. Everyone is scared *of* his first overnight pass. You'll find that it will be easier than you expect.
   B. It's understandable that you are concerned about your first night at home. Would it help if you make the decision after you've been home for a while and see how things are going?

C. I know how you feel, but the staff think that you are well enough to stay home overnight. Won't you try to do so?
D. It's important for you to try to remain at home overnight. If you are able to do it, it will be a measure of your improvement.

Questions 15-25.

DIRECTIONS: Questions 15 through 25 are to be answered on the basis of the following information.

Ms. Kathy Collins, 47 years old, has been hospitalized several times over a period of years because of episodes of elation and depression. She lives with her mother and sister. She is well known to the nursing staff. While she is again being admitted, she is chainsmoking cigarettes, walking back and forth, and talking loudly and gaily about her romantic successes.

15. Which of these greetings by the nurse who is admitting Ms. Collins would probably be MOST appropriate?

   A. We're sorry you had to come back, Ms. Collins, but we are glad to see you.
   B. Good morning, Ms. Collins. Your doctor called to say you were coming. I will show you to your room.
   C. Hello, Ms. Collins. You're cheerful this morning.
   D. It's good to see you again, Ms. Collins. You don't seem to mind coming back to the hospital.

15.____

16. The nurse who will care for Ms. Collins each day should expect to make use of which of these interventions?

   A. Distracting and redirecting
   B. Orienting and reminding
   C. Explaining and praising
   D. Evoking anger and encouraging insight

16.____

17. Ms. Collins is an overactive patient with a mood disturbance rather than a thought disorder.
Because of this type of illness, the nursing care plan should include measures that respond to the fact that she is

   A. disoriented
   B. easily stimulated by what is going on around her
   C. preoccupied with a single idea
   D. likely to be panicked by physical contact

17.____

18. Which of these nursing goals is likely to require the MOST attention while Ms. Collins is acutely ill?

   A. Orientation to time, place, and person
   B. Establishment of a sense of self-esteem
   C. Promotion of adequate rest
   D. Prevention of circulatory stasis

18.____

19. Ms. Collins and her roommate are in their room. While passing by, a registered nurse hears them arguing. Ms. Collins says, *You're a slob. How can anybody live in this mess!* The roommate answers, *What right do you have to say that?* and starts to cry.
Which of these interventions by the nurse would be appropriate?

    A. Enter the room and say to Ms. Collins, *You have upset your roommate. She's crying.*
    B. Enter and say, *It sounds as if you are both upset.*
    C. Stand in the doorway and say, *It's part of your therapy to learn how to get along together.*
    D. Take the roommate aside and explain to her that Ms. Collins can be expected to be difficult for a few days.

20. Ms. Collins is not eating sufficient food. Which approach by the nurse would probably be BEST as a first step in trying to get her to eat more?

    A. Giving her foods that she can eat with her fingers while she is moving about
    B. Conveying to her tactfully the idea that she has to eat
    C. Serving her food to her on a tray and telling her firmly but kindly to eat
    D. Assuring her that she can have anything she wants to eat whenever she wants it

21. The physician orders lithium carbonate for Ms. Collins. To accompany the order for lithium carbonate, the physician is likely to specify that

    A. the patient should lie down for a half hour after each dose
    B. the medication should be evenly distributed throughout each 24-hour period
    C. a salt-free diet should be provided for the patient
    D. the drug level of the patient's blood should be monitored regularly

22. When their desires are frustrated, patients such as Ms. Collins are likely to

    A. maintain a superficial affability
    B. sulk and retire temporarily from the situation
    C. suddenly show hostility and aggression
    D. seek support from personnel

23. Group psychotherapy is ordered for Ms. Collins. The CHIEF purpose of this therapy is to help her to

    A. socialize easily with a group
    B. gain self-knowledge through the sharing of problems
    C. identify various types of emotional problems and ways in which people handle them
    D. become acquainted with types of problems that will be encountered after discharge

24. After several days, Ms. Collins' behavior changes, and she becomes depressed. One night the nurse finds Ms. Collins unconscious in bed with a strip of her sheet tied around her neck. She is cyanotic and her respirations are labored and stertorous. After loosening the constriction around Ms. Collins' neck and signaling for help, which of these actions by the nurse would demonstrate the BEST judgment?

    A. Remain with her.
    B. Place her in the proper position and start artificial respiration.

C. Give her a vigorous thump on the sternum.
D. Raise the foot of her bed.

25. Ms. Collins is gradually improving, and the team talks of plans for her discharge. On a visit to the unit, Ms. Collins' mother and sister tell the nurse that Ms. Collins doesn't seem much better, and they are very hesitant about having her return home because of the previous problems they've had with her. Which of these actions should INITIALLY be taken by the nurse?

25.____

A. Suggest that the family find a place where Ms. Collins can live by herself after discharge.
B. Elaborate on Ms. Collins' hospital regimen and the normality of her present behavior.
C. Assure the relatives that Ms. Collins is better and refer them to the physician if they have further questions.
D. Listen to Ms. Collins' relatives and suggest that they make an appointment with the family counselor.

KEY (CORRECT ANSWERS)

1. B
2. D
3. C
4. B
5. A

6. D
7. B
8. C
9. C
10. D

11. A
12. B
13. C
14. B
15. B

16. A
17. B
18. C
19. B
20. A

21. D
22. C
23. B
24. A
25. D

EXAMINATION SECTION
TEST 1

DIRECTIONS: Each question or incomplete statement is followed by several suggested answers or completions. Select the one that BEST answers the question or completes the statement. *PRINT THE LETTER OF THE CORRECT ANSWER IN THE SPACE AT THE RIGHT.*

Questions 1-11.

DIRECTIONS: Questions 1 through 11 are to be answered on the basis of the following information.

Mike Douglas, a 46-year-old construction worker, is admitted to the hospital with deep lacerations of the arms and legs that resulted from a fall on his job. After surgery, he develops septicemia and is put on isolation.

1. Mr. Douglas' primary nurse, Tina, recognizes that clients on prolonged isolation with little sensory stimuli will MOST likely initially develop

    A. aggressive and acting-out behavior
    B. an attitude of indifference
    C. fantasies that replace realities
    D. many somatic complaints

2. Which action should the nurse take FIRST to show acceptance of Mr. Douglas and his needs?

    A. Support Mr. Douglas's positive adaptations to his limitations.
    B. Anticipate and meet Mr. Douglas's dependency needs.
    C. Encourage Mr. Douglas to express all of his feelings.
    D. Express to Mr. Douglas how difficult it must be for him.

3. Tina plans daily scheduled visits with Mr. Douglas.
During the introductory phase of the nurse-client relationship, the nurse should focus the communication on

    A. a definite goal that both have agreed on
    B. the happenings on the unit during the day
    C. any topic the client wants to talk about
    D. the client's past experiences with his family

4. Tina arranges her chair so that when she is seated she is facing Mr. Douglas. This position provides the MOST therapeutic seating arrangement because

    A. the nurse and Mr. Douglas will have better eye contact and observation
    B. the nurse can best convey a feeling of acceptance
    C. Mr. Douglas will be more relaxed and comfortable
    D. Mr. Douglas and the nurse will know this is not a social visit

5. Tina can BEST show that she is paying close attention to what Mr. Douglas is saying if she sits at eye level with Mr. Douglas and

   A. maintains eye contact with him
   B. keeps a social distance from him
   C. holds his hand
   D. leans toward him

6. Tina conveys to Mr. Douglas that the climate of their nurse-client relationship is a therapeutic one.
   This tone is basic to therapy because

   A. the nurse will be more therapeutic
   B. the client feels safe
   C. disturbances are eliminated
   D. the client is sick

7. The nurse should expect Mr. Douglas to communicate more readily when he is talking about his

   A. feelings about the hospitalization
   B. activities on the unit
   C. family and their relationship
   D. educational and occupational skills

8. During the therapeutic session with Mr. Douglas, it is MOST important that the nurse

   A. listen and assimilate pertinent information
   B. change the subject when the client is anxious
   C. remain neutral by not giving an opinion
   D. always refer problem areas back to the client

9. Mr. Douglas appears uncomfortable with periods of silence. What should Tina say to break the silence?

   A. Is there anything I can do for you?
   B. Are you ready to start talking again?
   C. It is helpful to think things over for a while.
   D. I think I must be upsetting you.

10. In terminating the nurse-client relationship with Mr. Douglas, Tina must plan for him to

    A. feel that he can depend on the nurse if there is another crisis
    B. become involved in group therapy after discharge
    C. transfer feelings of trust to others on the unit
    D. talk about the separation and his feelings regarding it

11. Tina should expect Mr. Douglas to be able to accomplish which goal in terminating the nurse-client relationship? He should

    A. be pleased with the relationship and wish to continue
    B. be satisfied, and able to handle his own health problems
    C. be relieved because he knows he can now depend on the nurse
    D. have decreased symptoms and make fewer demands

Questions 12-15.

DIRECTIONS: Questions 12 through 15 are to be answered on the basis of the following information.

Mr. Burlington was admitted to the hospital with a diagnosis of emphysema. He has been designated by the staff as a *troublemaker*. He constantly demands attention and criticizes everything that is done for him.

12. His primary nurse has never met Mr. Burlington. Upon entering his room for the first time, she hears him say, *I don't need a stranger to help me; I need special care.*
    Which assessment would be MOST correct?   12.____

    A. He does require special care.
    B. He does not like strangers to care for him.
    C. He needs someone who understands him.
    D. The staff is correct; he is a troublemaker.

13. The nurse tells Mr. Burlington that she would like to get to know him better before they make a plan of care. He replies, *My life is an open book; you can have all my history at the nurses' station.*
    Which analysis would be MOST correct at this time?   13.____

    A. The nurse has to know Mr. Burlington better before making an analysis.
    B. The nurse and Mr. Burlington should not work on a plan.
    C. Mr. Burlington's needs are in his medical history file.
    D. Mr. Burlington should be helped to identify his problems more appropriately.

14. Later, Mr. Burlington reports that he has always been afraid of being dependent on others. He states that he has always been his *own man*.
    Which would be the BEST reply to help him with a plan that would meet his dependent needs?   14.____

    A. Although you are dependent on us now, you will soon be on your own.
    B. You will still be independent although some adjustments will have to be made.
    C. There are times when we all have to be dependent on others.
    D. How do you feel when you have to depend on others?

15. Mr. Burlington and the nurse plan for him to express his emotions more appropriately. Which action by the client would indicate that he is implementing this plan?   15.____

    A. Recognizing the cause when he is upset with others
    B. Telling the staff that he is sorry for his previous behavior
    C. Taking a stand and telling others he can care for himself
    D. Arranging for a time with the staff when he can express his feelings freely

Questions 16-23.

DIRECTIONS: Questions 16 through 23 are to be answered on the basis of the following information.

Mr. Washington, who is 65 years old and has recently retired, is admitted to the hospital after complaining of constipation, nausea, vomiting, weakness, and general malaise.

Although all tests are negative for any physical disorder, Mr. Washington continues to think he is very ill.

16. Frank is Mr. Washington's primary nurse. When he enters Mr. Washington's room, he feels that his client is upset.
    How should the nurse greet Mr. Washington?

    A. How are you feeling this morning?
    B. I have a feeling that you have a problem.
    C. How did you sleep last night?
    D. I would like to know what is on your mind.

17. To prolong his wife's visits, Mr. Washington makes increasing demands on her and plays on her guilt feelings. Frank should intervene by

    A. determining what visiting hours would be the most beneficial
    B. explaining to Mr. Washington why he should be more considerate
    C. talking to Mrs. Washington about her feelings concerning her husband's hospitalization
    D. encouraging Mrs. Washington to stay as long as her husband wants her to

18. Mr. Washington tells the nurse that he has never had an angry feeling toward his wife. The nurse recognizes this statement as a defensive reaction of denial, which is

    A. developing the opposite attitude to the way he is feeling
    B. rejecting something that is very disturbing to him
    C. giving a logical reason for something he wants to happen
    D. keeping his unacceptable experiences in his unconscious mind

19. Mr. Washington is constantly demanding attention. Even after his call bell is answered, he buzzes the nurses' station again.
    Which action by the nurse is MOST therapeutic?

    A. Refer Mr. Washington to a mental health counselor for consultation.
    B. Assist Mr. Washington to see himself as others see him.
    C. Orient Mr. Washington to the hospital policy of client involvement.
    D. Talk to Mr. Washington because he needs to discuss his fears.

20. When Mr. Washington starts treating Frank as if he were his son, the nurse should understand that the client is

    A. anticipating the roles that he and the nurse will play
    B. acting this way so that they will have a deeper relationship
    C. reacting to the way the nurse has treated him
    D. using a fantasy relationship when dealing with reality

21. Frank recognizes that Mr. Washington's covert behavior is difficult to identify because covert behavior

    A. is so obvious that it is taken for granted
    B. is so subtle that it cannot be perceived
    C. is obscured by defenses in adults
    D. seldom appears in an adult's reaction

22. Mr. Washington tells Frank, *I have something important to tell you, but you must promise you won't tell anyone else.* The nurse should understand that Mr. Washington is

    A. anxious to share his feelings with the nurse
    B. testing the reliability of the nurse
    C. showing his faith in the nurse
    D. conveying that he is afraid of exposure

22.____

23. How should Frank answer Mr. Washington's request for complete confidentiality?

    A. I think you shouldn't tell me if you are not sure.
    B. To provide continuity of care, I will have to tell the staff.
    C. If it is that important, I won't tell anyone.
    D. Let's discuss your need to tell only me.

23.____

Questions 24-30.

DIRECTIONS: Questions 24 through 30 are to be answered on the basis of the following information.

Four nurses are assigned to the day care of the 28 clients on an acute care mental health unit in the general hospital. Each nurse acts as a primary nurse for seven clients.

24. The staff meets twice a week to discuss which environment would be the most therapeutic for their clients.
Which principle should be basic to ALL of their decisions concerning the clients' environment?

    A. The environment must be as nearly like the client's home as possible.
    B. The client must have a voice in the decision-making process.
    C. Sufficient care must be provided in the least restrictive environment.
    D. Each environment must provide psychotherapy and medical supervision.

24.____

25. The staff discusses telling the clients their rights upon admission to the hospital. The value of these rights is to

    A. make clients aware of what their responsibilities are when hospitalized
    B. let clients know that they have the right to leave
    C. provide rules so the staff will not neglect their clients while giving care
    D. provide clients with laws that will influence their care

25.____

26. The staff on the mental health unit has a philosophy of critical timing for nursing intervention. This means that the staff feels that this period is critical to the outcome of the client's treatment.
What period of time would this be?

    A. The first month of working in groups
    B. Within one week of a one-to-one relationship
    C. Within 2 months of hospitalization
    D. The first 24 hours after admission

26.____

27. It is MOST important that the nursing staff in a mental health unit make an overall psychosocial assessment and treatment plan for each client because

   A. it is the legal contract of the nursing approach to the client's care
   B. it provides the client with documentation of the nursing approach
   C. there will be a unified approach to the client
   D. the nursing goals are specifically related to the client's needs

28. The staff discusses the nurse's liability for clients who are out of control.
Which action by the nurse would make him or her liable for a battery indictment?

   A. Restraining the client from harming others on the unit
   B. Threatening the client physically if he or she does not behave
   C. Putting the client on isolation until control is gained
   D. Restraining the client after he has gained control as a precautionary measure

29. The recording of a crisis episode and the nursing intervention provided on a client's chart is essential for the protection of the client and the nurse.
Which of the following is the MOST accurate recording of the crisis and treatment process?

   A. After visit with family, client was extremely depressed. Nursing staff notified.
   B. Family visits apparently depressed client. Spoke of *wanting to end it all.* Placed on 15 minute check.
   C. Client stated, *I want to end it all.* Dr. John alerted. Assigned 24-hour nursing observation.
   D. Client spoke of suicide and was placed on suicidal precautions.

30. In planning for the client's discharge from the mental health unit, which action by the professional staff is IMPERATIVE?

   A. Medical supervision of the client to provide adequate psychotropic medication
   B. Adequate aftercare by a professional group that will ensure stabilization in the community
   C. Assurance that the client has someone in the community who will be responsible for him or her
   D. Assurance that the client will not harm himself or other people in the community

KEY (CORRECT ANSWERS)

1.	C	16.	B
2.	D	17.	C
3.	C	18.	B
4.	A	19.	D
5.	D	20.	A
6.	B	21.	C
7.	B	22.	B
8.	A	23.	D
9.	C	24.	C
10.	D	25.	D
11.	B	26.	D
12.	C	27.	A
13.	D	28.	D
14.	D	29.	C
15.	A	30.	B

TEST 2

DIRECTIONS: Each question or incomplete statement is followed by several suggested answers or completions. Select the one that BEST answers the question or completes the statement. *PRINT THE LETTER OF THE CORRECT ANSWER IN THE SPACE AT THE RIGHT.*

Questions 1-11.

DIRECTIONS: Questions 1 through 11 are to be answered on the basis of the following information.

    Monica Smith, age 24, is an unmarried woman who lives with her mother, sister, and brother in a private residence. She is attending the neurological outpatient clinic for the first time. She has a history of two grand mal seizures.

    A diagnosis of idiopathic epilepsy has been made. The physician has ordered an electroencephalogram (EEG) and phenytoin sodium (dilantin), 300 mg/day.

1. Monica's second, and most recent, seizure was a grand mal seizure. The nurses recognized that the seizure was *grand mal* because

    A. petit mal seizures do not recur
    B. she suffered amnesia
    C. she had mild twitching and jerking motions
    D. she remained conscious

1.___

2. While taking Monica's history, the nurse should recognize that

    A. grand mal seizures do not cause mental deterioration
    B. idiopathic epilepsy is a form of mental illness
    C. idiopathic epilepsy lowers intelligence level
    D. a common characteristic of idiopathic epilepsy is committing violent acts

2.___

3. To prepare Monica for the EEG, the nurse should explain to her that

    A. the test measures mental status as well as electrical brain waves
    B. she will be unconscious during the test and will feel no pain
    C. during the test she will experience slight electric shocks that feel like pin pricks
    D. it is a painless procedure which measures the brain's electrical activity

3.___

4. Health teaching for Monica includes ensuring that she understands that

    A. forcing fluids helps reduce the incidence of seizures
    B. the incidence of seizures is related to hyperglycemia
    C. proper prophylactic medication can control the incidence of seizures
    D. use of alcoholic beverages, in moderation, is permitted

4.___

5. During a follow-up clinic visit, Monica tells the nurse that her urine has had a reddish-brown color.
The nurse should

5.___

A. notify the physician that Monica has hematuria
B. tell Monica that this is a sign of hepatic toxicity
C. reassure Monica that this is a harmless side effect of phenytoin sodium
D. recommend to Monica that she go to the laboratory for a serum dilantin concentration test

6. A long-term goal for Monica is to minimize the gingival hyperplasia associated with dilantin therapy.
The nurse should recognize that

A. a regular plan of good oral hygiene is essential
B. the physician will reduce the dosage at the first sign of hyperplasia
C. vitamin C should be taken daily with the dilantin
D. another anticonvulsant will be prescribed if it occurs

6._____

7. Monica's serum concentration level of dilantin is 15 µg/ml. The nurse should recognize this as _____ serum level.

A. a toxic
B. below the desired therapeutic
C. above the recommended
D. a desired therapeutic

7._____

8. Family members should be instructed about caring for Monica during a grand mal seizure.
IMMEDIATE care during a seizure should include

A. giving a vitamin C rich juice before the clonic stage begins
B. turning Monica's head to the side
C. restraining Monica's arms and legs
D. forcing the mouth open to insert an airway

8._____

9. The nurse explains to Monica that safety precautions can be taken by those who have warning symptoms before the seizure.
What warning symptoms should the nurse tell Monica to be aware of?

A. Tingling in a local region, anxiety, and lack of consciousness
B. Increased toxicity of muscles and autonomic behavior
C. Hot and cold sensations, gastrointestinal problems, anxiety, and mood changes
D. Muscle twitching, lapse of consciousness, and anxiety

9._____

10. The nurse should tell Monica's family that after a seizure she will be in a confused state and will need some supervision.
It is MOST important for the caregiver to be calm, because the confused state of the epileptic is considered to be a(n)

A. gross impairment in social and intellectual functioning with crude, tactless, and impulsive behavior
B. helpless state, with intellectual deterioration and regression to the infantile state
C. feeling of general inadequacy and fatigue that results in a decrease of interest
D. adaptive period, when one slowly learns to cope with the devastating insults to one's psychological and physical integrity

10._____

11. Monica asks the nurse if it is true that there is an *epileptic personality*. What is the nurse's BEST response?

    A. The person may take on a sick role if mismanaged at home or in the community.
    B. Be aware that anxiety over anticipation of a seizure may cause personality problems.
    C. Yes, one may learn to induce seizures as a way of getting attention from others.
    D. No, deviation in personality is caused by restrictions imposed by society.

Questions 12-20.

DIRECTIONS: Questions 12 through 20 are to be answered on the basis of the following information.

Phillip Wright, 36 years old, is admitted to the mental health unit after taking an overdose of phenobarbital. He is assigned to nurse Beth for primary care. He tells her that, although he is a very successful lawyer and happily married with two children, he has been depressed for about 4 months and does not know why.

12. Which nursing diagnosis would BEST identify Mr. Wright's problem?

    A. Altered thought processes
    B. Ineffective individual coping
    C. Sensory/perceptual alterations
    D. Potential for injury

13. The nurse observes that Mr. Wright's facial expression and responses are those of a deeply depressed person.
His facial expression is _____, and his responses are_____.

    A. frightened; angry
    B. anxious; tense
    C. resigned; fearful
    D. mournful; monotonous

14. Mrs. Wright asks the nurse if there were symptoms that her husband was depressed even before he appeared that way.
The nurse should reply that the EARLY signs and symptoms of depression include

    A. poor appetite and sleep disturbances
    B. hypermobility and increased speech pattern
    C. unsteady gait and a mask-like expression
    D. complaints of somatic pains and weakness

15. Mr. Wright has been placed on a *suicide watch* by the mental health team. Which plan would offer the BEST protection for Mr. Wright?

    A. Securing the unit with locked doors and barred windows
    B. A relaxed and accepting environment
    C. Having a staff member stay with him at all times
    D. Restricting the use of belts, glassware, or sharp instruments

16. In planning nursing care for Mr. Wright, the MOST therapeutic approach would be

    A. showing sympathy for his suffering and deep depression
    B. remaining neutral and showing him respect

C. speaking of pleasant things to cheer him up
D. reflecting his feelings by speaking in a sorrowful tone

17. Mr. Wright does not talk unless spoken to during his therapeutic sessions with the nurse. Which would be the BEST nursing intervention?

    A. Leave him alone until he feels more at ease
    B. Sit with him but remain silent until he speaks
    C. Continue talking to him to encourage his participation
    D. Arrange to have him involved in social activities

18. Mr. Wright says he cannot participate in any activities because he finds it difficult to concentrate.
    The MOST therapeutic response by the nurse would be:

    A. You will not be expected to participate until you are ready
    B. Activity is necessary for you to work off your pent-up emotions
    C. You will never know what you can do until you try it
    D. The choice is not up to you because it is the staff that arranges the schedule

19. Which nursing intervention would BEST help Mr. Wright to cope with his feelings of depression?

    A. Suggest that he become more involved in outside activities
    B. Interrupt his feelings and focus on something more realistic
    C. Discuss his ambivalence, disappointments, and resentments with him
    D. Encourage him to talk of his depression and guilt feelings

20. When Mr. Wright is discharged, the MOST important follow-up care would be

    A. referral to community resources
    B. education for socialization
    C. crisis intervention
    D. group participation

Questions 21-25.

DIRECTIONS: Questions 21 through 25 are to be answered on the basis of the following information.

David Rodriguez is a 34-year-old lawyer who has been hospitalized with a severe anxiety attack.

21. The nurse plans to help Mr. Rodriguez become desensitized to his neurotic attachment to anxiety.
    Which approach would be the MOST therapeutic?

    A. Talk to him about his feelings when he is feeling very anxious
    B. Sit quietly with him when he is anxious, until he relaxes
    C. Get him busy doing something when he is very anxious
    D. Support him while he endures planned-for increased anxiety

22. While caring for Mr. Rodriguez, the nurse should especially try to intervene whenever he is observed as being

    A. accepting of different kinds of behavior
    B. outgoing and assertive
    C. overconscientious and/or rigid
    D. uncomfortable in a family situation

23. Mr. Rodriguez tells the nurse he cannot participate in any social activities because he gets very anxious.
Which would be the nurse's BEST reply?

    A. The time has come for you to assume some responsibility.
    B. I'm sorry you're not well; tell me about it.
    C. It is a rule of the unit; all must participate.
    D. I will go with you, but participation is up to you.

24. Mr. Rodriguez seems more anxious after seeing his psychiatrist. He tells the nurse that the sessions with the doctor always make him feel more anxious.
The nurse's BEST reply would be:

    A. The doctor and I both understand this is a trying time for you
    B. The doctor's aim is to help you, not make you feel worse
    C. This always happens at the beginning; you will feel better
    D. Therapy helps one to have insight, and this can be uncomfortable

25. Anxiety is a result of

    A. elevated blood pressure
    B. the anticipation of danger or failure
    C. a consciously recognized, external threat or danger
    D. drug withdrawal

Questions 26-30.

    DIRECTIONS: In Questions 26 through 30, match the numbered symptom or reaction to the lettered disorder, listed in the column below, to which it is MOST closely related.

        A. Phobia
        B. Agoraphobia
        C. Obsessive compulsive disorder
        D. Anxiety
        E. Post traumatic stress disorder

26. Denial

27. Reaction formation

28. Projection

29. Symbolization

30. Regression

KEY (CORRECT ANSWERS)

1.	B	16.	B
2.	A	17.	C
3.	D	18.	B
4.	C	19.	C
5.	C	20.	A
6.	A	21.	D
7.	D	22.	C
8.	B	23.	D
9.	C	24.	D
10.	D	25.	B
11.	A	26.	E
12.	B	27.	C
13.	D	28.	B
14.	A	29.	A
15.	C	30.	D

EXAMINATION SECTION
TEST 1

DIRECTIONS: Each question or incomplete statement is followed by several suggested answers or completions. Select the one that BEST answers the question or completes the statement. *PRINT THE LETTER OF THE CORRECT ANSWER IN THE SPACE AT THE RIGHT.*

Questions 1-13.

DIRECTIONS: Questions 1 through 13 are to be answered on the basis of the following information.

Sonny Burnett, a drug addict, is admitted to the hospital and is suspected of having hepatitis. The diagnosis of Type B hepatitis is confirmed, and Sonny is placed in a unit with other drug addicts. A decision to attempt a *cold turkey* withdrawal for Sonny is made by the health team.

1. Which of the following observations indicates that Sonny has recently had *a fix?*

    A. Increased blood pressure
    B. Fruity breath
    C. Needle marks on his extremities
    D. Constricted pupils

2. Which of the following statements should be included in the nurse's instructions to Sonny concerning his illness?

    A. Treatment with hepatitis B immune globulin will provide you with immunity.
    B. You have developed an immunity to viral hepatitis.
    C. You will have a lifelong immunity to serum hepatitis.
    D. You will always be more susceptible to serum hepatitis.

3. To prevent the spread of the disease to others, the nurse should place Sonny on _____ isolation precautions.

    A. blood and body fluids
    B. respiratory and body fluids
    C. respiratory and enteric
    D. enteric and blood

4. The nursing care plan includes expanding the range of interests of the clients in Sonny's group.
   The MOST therapeutic initial approach would be to

    A. accept the group's need to communicate in the addict's jargon
    B. speak to the group about the harmful effects of drug abuse
    C. support the group members in their need to discuss their habit
    D. discourage the group from discussing drugs or having gutter talk

5. The symptoms that Sonny would MOST likely exhibit at the onset of *cold turkey* withdrawal are

   A. weight loss, severe stomach cramps, and vomiting
   B. muscular pain, anorexia, and diarrhea
   C. diaphoresis, yawning, lacrimation, and sneezing
   D. restlessness, insomnia, and increased blood pressure

6. Sonny asks the nurse how long he is going to suffer the withdrawal symptoms. The MOST accurate reply by the nurse would be that if you just started withdrawal, symptoms should begin in _____ hours, peak in _____, and subside in _____.

   A. 4; 24 hours; 48 hours
   B. 12; 36 hours; 72 hours
   C. 24; 3 days; 5 days
   D. 36; 5 days; 7 days

7. The MOST therapeutic action by the nurse during the peak phase of Sonny's withdrawal from heroin would be

   A. providing adequate fluid intake
   B. providing a supplementary diet
   C. instituting convulsion precautions
   D. administering prescribed sedation

8. Sonny's laboratory findings show a slight improvement, but he is suffering from appetite loss.
   To ensure adequate nutrition, the nurse should

   A. request an order for intravenous fluid and vitamin therapy
   B. weigh Sonny at least every second day and keep him informed of his weight changes
   C. provide Sonny with small meals and high-protein beverages between meals
   D. encourage ambulation to stimulate Sonny's appetite

9. Sonny was found with the following symptoms during his withdrawal from heroin. Which set of symptoms suggests a complication that would require IMMEDIATE nursing intervention?

   A. Marked rise in temperature or blood pressure, or both
   B. Anxiety, tremors, and depression
   C. Nausea, vomiting, and diarrhea
   D. Profuse diaphoresis, influenza symptoms, and chills

10. Sonny and the health care team discuss what type of environment he needs for best recovery from his drug problem and decide on a structured environment.
    Of the following characteristics of this environment, the one that will be of GREATEST basic benefit to Sonny is

    A. having others tell him what to do
    B. knowing what the rules are and what is expected of him
    C. being protected from outside influences
    D. learning more about the effects of drugs

11. Sonny, after noticing and being curious, asks the nurse why some of the clients are receiving methadone as a replacement for heroin.
    The BEST reply by the nurse would be that this narcotic is given because it

    A. cannot be taken with other drugs
    B. is nonaddictive
    C. gives a euphoric feeling
    D. relieves withdrawal symptoms

11.____

12. Sonny asks the nurse why it is necessary for one to have a periodic urine test when taking methadone.
    Which of the following would be the BEST reply by the nurse?

    A. We need to test the kidneys' threshold to methadone.
    B. Methadone irritates the kidneys, so we have to do a kidney function test.
    C. We test for drugs other than methadone.
    D. We have to determine the methadone dosage.

12.____

13. Sonny wants to know why heroin causes hepatitis.
    The explanation by the nurse that would be MOST appropriate for Sonny is:

    A. Heroin reduces one's natural defenses
    B. Hepatitis is not caused by heroin
    C. Hepatitis is caused by a germ found on the skin
    D. Hepatitis is caused by using dirty needles

13.____

Questions 14-18.

DIRECTIONS: Questions 14 through 18 are to be answered on the basis of the following information.

Linda Carter, age 24, just got discharged from the hospital after being treated for substance abuse. She is addicted to alcohol and cocaine. She is now seeing Ms. Flores, the nurse at the local mental health center.

14. Ms. Flores plans to help Linda adjust to the activities of the community mental health center.
    The FIRST action taken by the nurse should be to

    A. ask for a detailed history of threatened drug abuse
    B. assess her own feelings about the client's lack of control
    C. assign the client to a volunteer who also has had a drug problem
    D. introduce herself and state her objectives

14.____

15. Linda tells the group at the health center that her drinking was caused by her family, who all drank like fish. How should the nurse analyze this behavior?

    A. Linda's family was the cause of her drug use.
    B. Most users get addicted to drugs through their families.
    C. The behavior of most drug users is aggression turned outward.
    D. Linda does not take responsibility for her drug use.

15.____

16. Linda comes to the center with alcohol odor on her breath. The nurse should 16.____

    A. assign her to an Alcoholics Anonymous group meeting
    B. call her family to come and take her home
    C. ask her what happened to make her want a drink
    D. tell her that she cannot come to the center while drinking

17. Linda tells the nurse that she always felt she wasn't good enough, and with drugs she felt 17.____
    she was the greatest. The BEST plan of action for her at this time would be to

    A. suggest that she put trust in a supreme being
    B. offer recognition for accomplishing tasks
    C. encourage her to talk to others who have similar problems
    D. recommend that she live life one day at a time

18. Another important plan for the future that Linda and the nurse should make to help her 18.____
    overcome her addictive behavior is that she must

    A. not resume a relationship with her old drinking friends
    B. find a time-filling and gratifying occupation
    C. not attend any social gatherings without a chaperone
    D. move back into the protective environment of her family

Questions 19-28.

DIRECTIONS: Questions 19 through 28 are to be answered on the basis of the following information.

Burt Right, 28 years old, has a history of juvenile offenses, having an arrogant manner, always being a loner, and preferring to do things his own way. He can see no wrong in himself and no right in others.

Due to his aggressive behavior, he once got involved in a serious fight and got shot in the right leg. While Burt's physical condition has been improving, he continually demonstrates disruptive behavior. He has been arrogant and demanding.

19. After a psychiatric consultation, Burt is diagnosed as having antisocial behavior. 19.____
    Which problem exhibited by the client would be the MOST difficult for the staff to handle?

    A. Having problems in distinguishing true statements from lies
    B. Not being able to form a close relationship
    C. Being persistent in his antisocial behavior
    D. Not learning from experience

20. Burt is transferred to a psychiatric unit. During orientation, Burt is told of the rules and 20.____
    regulations of the unit. One day, he borrows another person's shampoo without permission. He says to the nurse, *It's not stealing when you borrow shampoo.*
    The nurse's BEST response in this situation is:

    A. Keep the shampoo; I will get more for the other patient.
    B. Give the client his shampoo back and tell him you are sorry

C. You will not be penalized; the rules do not include borrowing shampoo
D. The rule is, when you steal you will be penalized

21. When Burt is confronted about his unacceptable behavior toward others, the staff should expect him to

    A. become very angry
    B. accept the criticism
    C. show very little concern
    D. withdraw from others

22. The group which would probably provide the MOST therapeutic advice in the course of determining penalties for breaking the rules of the mental health unit would be the

    A. clients who live in the unit and have to abide by the rules
    B. lay people in the community who determine hospital policy
    C. members of the administrative group who determine the rules of the hospital
    D. members of the mental health professional staff who set the standards of the unit

23. Which approach by the nursing team would be MOST effective with Burt?

    A. Providing a nonstructured environment
    B. Being a part of the therapeutic community
    C. A one-to-one relationship
    D. Allowing Burt to direct his treatment

24. Burt appears to be very reliable, has excellent reasoning, is not reacting in an emotionally disturbed way, and his actions seem to be completely normal.
    The nurse can BEST assess his behavior through obtaining

    A. Burt's cooperation and consent
    B. a series of psychological tests
    C. a detailed history from Burt
    D. his behavioral history from acquaintances

25. The health team has been observing Burt's interactions with members of his family. Which behavior of the family would MOST likely contribute to Burt's illness?

    A. Being overprotective, hypochondriacal, symbiotic, and dependent
    B. Violence, indifference, rejection, and lack of predictability
    C. Using sexual provocation and being compulsive and rigid
    D. Setting goals too high, and thus making Burt feel guilty

26. The members of the staff have started having difficulty accepting Burt and have started criticizing him even when he has not broken a rule.
    The PROBABLE reason for this nontherapeutic approach is that

    A. Burt's behavior is very destructive to others
    B. Burt's behavior is considered pathological
    C. Burt does not reinforce the staff for its efforts
    D. the staff can show Burt that inconsistency is not therapeutic

27. The nurse analyzing Burt's behavior recognizes that he is often in conflict with others because he has

   A. disguised his deep feelings for others
   B. never learned group norms and loyalty
   C. reverted to regressive patterns of behavior
   D. lived his life in an asocial environment

28. Burt and his family have been in therapy for eight months. Burt is receiving therapy through the hospital clinic.
   In evaluating Burt's progress, the health team is most likely to observe that Burt shows internalized acceptable behavior MOST often

   A. when interacting with the clients
   B. after talking to the nursing staff
   C. after visits with his family
   D. during the hourly sessions with his doctor

Questions 29-30.

DIRECTIONS: Questions 29 and 30 are to be answered on the basis of the following information.

A client of yours is Jill Lebensfield, who is 30 years old. She was admitted because she had attacked her neighbor with a knife as, according to her, the neighbor was unlawfully wiretapping her house. She continues to feel that others are spying on her.

29. Jill tells the nurse, *I'm not crazy; I don't belong here, my neighbor does.*
   What behavior pattern is she using?

   A. Sociopathic   B. Aggressive
   C. Neurotic   D. Projective

30. Jill uses this behavior because

   A. she never learned to control her temper
   B. it is a secondary gain of aggressive behavior
   C. some aspects of her life are difficult to handle
   D. social-moral codes were never learned

KEY (CORRECT ANSWERS)

1.	D	16.	C
2.	C	17.	B
3.	A	18.	A
4.	D	19.	D
5.	C	20.	D
6.	B	21.	C
7.	A	22.	A
8.	C	23.	B
9.	A	24.	D
10.	B	25.	B
11.	D	26.	C
12.	C	27.	B
13.	D	28.	A
14.	B	29.	D
15.	D	30.	C

TEST 2

DIRECTIONS: Each question or incomplete statement is followed by several suggested answers or completions. Select the one that BEST answers the question or completes the statement. *PRINT THE LETTER OF THE CORRECT ANSWER IN THE SPACE AT THE RIGHT.*

Questions 1-11.

DIRECTIONS: Questions 1 through 11 are to be answered on the basis of the following information.

Norman Bates, 24 years old, is brought to the emergency mental health center by his family. He had furiously tried to attack his mother. For the last 6 months, since graduating from college, he has not been able to find employment, and most of the time he sits and stares into space. On admission, he appears dazed and speaks incoherently.

1. The nurse observes that Mr. Bates sits alone in the dayroom staring at the floor. His clothes are disheveled, and his hair and beard are unkempt. She approaches him and introduces herself as his primary nurse.
   Which statement would be MOST appropriate by the nurse at this time?

   A. There is a meeting of all new clients and I will introduce you.
   B. I will sit with you for 10 minutes. You don't have to talk.
   C. This is the hour for occupational therapy. I will go with you.
   D. If you care to, you may go to your room. You had a difficult night.

2. The nurse observes Mr. Bates sitting alone. He is staring into space, smiling, and moving his lips as if talking to someone.
   How should the nurse approach him?

   A. What do you see when you stare into space?
   B. You must not sit by yourself; you will hear voices.
   C. Tell me what the voices are telling you.
   D. You were moving your lips, but made no sound.

3. Mr. Bates tells the nurse that he hears voices telling him he is a good person.
   The MOST accurate reply by the nurse would be:

   A. A stimulating environment can enhance one's senses and cause hallucinations.
   B. You have an overactive imagination that makes up for a dull existence.
   C. There are unconscious feelings breaking into your consciousness.
   D. There must be some pathology to the sensory organ receptors or nerves.

4. Mr. Bates asks the nurse when the best time to try to control the voices would be.
   Which reply would be MOST accurate?
   _____ the voices.

   A. When you are actively hearing
   B. When you are not hearing
   C. When you are waiting to hear
   D. Immediately after hearing

5. Mr. Bates tells the nurse, *You have a time to contact the individual.* The nurse recognizes that this is speech that has meaning only for the client in his primitive thoughts. What type of speech is this?

   A. Word salad
   B. Magical thinking
   C. Looseness of association
   D. Neologisms

6. Mr. Bates asks the nurse to give him an example of his behavior that the doctor called *delusions of reference*. Which reply by the nurse would be ACCURATE?

   A. The room is wired by the police, who want to get me.
   B. My body is disintegrating into a mass of jelly.
   C. I'm the prince of Wales; my name is Charles.
   D. The conversations and actions of others are always concerning me.

7. The nurse tells Mr. Bates that the long-term goal for the nurse/client therapeutic sessions is to help him

   A. accept his behavior and not feel guilty
   B. learn to communicate in a less symbolic way
   C. understand the reason for his sick behavior
   D. learn new skills so that he can find employment

8. After several weeks of daily therapeutic sessions, Mr. Bates tells the nurse, *You are like everyone else; you don't understand me – you are pushing.*
   How should the nurse reply?

   A. Do you feel that I have been pushing you too fast?
   B. Not being understood must be very difficult.
   C. Who is this everyone else I remind you of?
   D. Maybe we should find someone else to replace me.

9. Mr. Bates asks the nurse why so many clients return to the hospital after being discharged.
   The MAIN reason for this revolving-door syndrome is

   A. families and the community reject the client
   B. the client refuses to return for follow-up care in the community
   C. the client cannot find suitable employment
   D. a symbiotic relationship has developed with the staff

10. The nurse and Mr. Bates are ready to plan for his participation in groups.
    Before making this plan, it should be considered whether he

    A. is accepted by other clients on the unit
    B. is ready to be discharged from the hospital
    C. can tolerate the nurse without stress
    D. still needs the nurse's support

11. A week before his discharge, Mr. Bates and the nurse go on a shopping trip.
    The MAIN objective of this activity is to

    A. boost Mr. Bates' self-esteem by providing diversional activity in the community
    B. give Mr. Bates an opportunity to buy some clothes

C. assist Mr. Bates in implementing some skills he learned in the hospital
D. condition Mr. Bates toward acceptable behavior in the community

Questions 12-30.

DIRECTIONS: Questions 12 through 30 are to be answered on the basis of the following information.

Bobby Briggs, age 20, has been hospitalized for 14 days with compound fractures of the right tibia and fibula resulting from a motorcycle accident. After closed reduction of the fractures, he is placed in traction. His personality evaluation indicates that he is a shy, introspective person who keeps to himself and never talks unless asked a direct question. He has had no visitors.

12. Bobby's nurse assesses his emotional problem.
The nurse understands that, at his age, a PRIMARY developmental task is to

   A. have a sense of self and extended self in an intimate relationship
   B. seek to become a part of a group with a sense of belonging to this group
   C. have identified life's goals such as occupational and marital choices
   D. gain feelings of self-worth as a result of appraisals from significant others

13. The nurse observes that Bobby appears very insecure.
The MOST effective nursing action in helping to alleviate Bobby's insecurity would be to

   A. allow him freedom to do what he wants
   B. plan a consistent staff approach based on his needs
   C. provide for his physical and emotional needs
   D. assign someone to be with him until his anxiety subsides

14. The nurse understands that Bobby's withdrawn behavior is MOST likely due to the fact that

   A. there is a constant need for approval, yet he resents it
   B. he has identified with the parent who lacks superego control
   C. he has received too much protection from significant others
   D. interpersonal relationships become a source of anxiet

15. The nurse also understands that Bobby's behavior is a defense, because the world of reality is painful for him. Which behavior should the nurse observe to confirm this?

   A. He avoids relationships by staying at a safe and familiar level of functioning.
   B. His emotions have created visceral changes and he has repressed his emotions.
   C. He can admit no fault in himself or any virtue in others.
   D. He is preoccupied with a sense of self-deprecation and self-reproach.

16. The nurse has planned a series of interviews with Bobby.
The nurse should place the chair _____ from the client, to provide an appropriate space.

   A. 4 to 8 inches
   B. 8 to 24 inches
   C. 18 inches to 4 feet
   D. 4 to 8 feet

17. The nurse understands that at this distance the nurse and client are more comfortable because

    A. the voice can be kept at a whisper
    B. fine details of the other person are lost
    C. they can touch one another without reaching
    D. vision and perception are not distorted

17._____

18. The nurse makes an appointment with Bobby to talk to him daily for approximately 30 minutes.
    The nurse's PRIMARY goal in arranging these meetings is to

    A. aid Bobby with his socializing problem by socializing with him
    B. assist in identifying his problems in a one-to-one relationship
    C. help have a feeling that others in the environment care
    D. determine from Bobby why he is so withdrawn and has no friends

18._____

19. After being introduced, Bobby does not acknowledge the nurse's presence.
    The nurse should know that

    A. admission to a new environment causes him to withdraw
    B. he needs rest if proper healing is to take place
    C. the accident may also have caused some brain injury
    D. rejection of interpersonal relationships is part of his defense

19._____

20. The FIRST short-term goal for the nurse to establish as a nursing care need of Bobby should be to

    A. establish and maintain the client's contact with reality
    B. provide for trust and security in the nurse/client relationship
    C. initiate and develop the nurse/client relationship
    D. encourage and support the client's interactions with others

20._____

21. At an early session, Bobby complains of discomfort in his lower back.
    What action by the nurse would BEST meet Bobby's needs?

    A. Give him simple instructions for isometric exercises for the back.
    B. Give him his prn medication of Tylenol, 1000 mg.
    C. Give him a back rub while he raises his hip.
    D. Ask him when he had his last bowel movement.

21._____

22. The nurse implements nursing care to alleviate Bobby's back pain because

    A. physical touching will alleviate pain and also provide trust and security needed
    B. lack of bowel movement can cause pressure on the lower back
    C. isometric exercises will strengthen muscles and prevent atrophy
    D. Tylenol reduces pain caused by muscle spasms

22._____

23. Bobby tells the nurse that he has always liked to be alone. He states, *You know, the best company is my own.*
    Which reply by the nurse would BEST expand his experience?

    A. You have a great deal of self-confidence, don't you?
    B. Are you saying you never enjoy the company of others?

23._____

C. Tell me how it makes you feel to be with others.
D. You will miss a lot of life by being a loner.

24. Although Bobby answers direct questions, there are long periods of silence.
The nurse understands that Bobby is using this silence because he is

   A. thinking of what to say
   B. clarifying his thoughts
   C. severely depressed
   D. uncomfortable with others

25. The nurse can BEST break the silence with Bobby by saying:

   A. If I'm upsetting you, I'll be back later
   B. It must be difficult to talk to strangers
   C. What are you thinking about?
   D. Do these sessions with me make you nervous?

26. The nurse observes that Bobby cracks his knuckles whenever he is anxious. Which nursing action would be MOST therapeutic?

   A. Give him something to do with his hands so he will be occupied.
   B. Ask the physician to prescribe a mild tranquilizer for him.
   C. Explain to Bobby that this behavior will make his hands arthritic.
   D. Assess what causes this behavior and take steps to lessen his discomfort.

27. At another session, Bobby tells the nurse that his brother was to blame for the motorcycle accident. He states that if his brother hadn't sold it to him, he wouldn't be in this fix today.
The nurse understands that this statement reflects

   A. avoidance of a close relationship with his brother
   B. an impression that a different cycle would have been safer
   C. dislike of his brother who sold a defective cycle
   D. feelings of failure that he attributes to his brother

28. After Bobby made the statement blaming his brother for the accident, the nurse should reply:

   A. What do you and your family do for pleasure when you are together?
   B. This must be a difficult time for you. How did the accident happen?
   C. You feel that your brother sold you an inferior bike.
   D. It must be difficult for you being in pain, while your brother is not.

29. Bobby's health condition has improved.
The observation by the nurse that indicates that Bobby's emotional health has also improved is that he

   A. is able to talk about his problem and not withdraw
   B. gives the staff a box of chocolate for helping him
   C. tells the nurse he can work on his problems alone
   D. discontinues the sessions with the nurse therapist

30. Which referral group would be MOST beneficial for Bobby at the time he leaves the hospital? 30._____

    A. Group of people who have problems communicating
    B. Safety driving school for motorcyclists
    C. Public health department for follow-up care
    D. Encounter group where Bobby will be forced to look at his behavior

KEY (CORRECT ANSWERS)

1.	D	16.	C
2.	B	17.	D
3.	C	18.	B
4.	C	19.	D
5.	A	20.	C
6.	D	21.	C
7.	B	22.	A
8.	C	23.	C
9.	B	24.	D
10.	C	25.	B
11.	D	26.	D
12.	A	27.	D
13.	B	28.	B
14.	D	29.	A
15.	A	30.	C

www.ingramcontent.com/pod-product-compliance
Lightning Source LLC
Chambersburg PA
CBHW081807300426
44116CB00014B/2271